Person Centred Practice for Professionals

Person Centred Practice for Professionals

Edited by Jeanette Thompson,
Jackie Kilbane and Helen Sanderson

 Open University Press

Open University Press
McGraw-Hill Education
McGraw-Hill House
Shoppenhangers Road
Maidenhead
Berkshire
England
SL6 2QL

email: enquiries@openup.co.uk
world wide web: www.openup.co.uk

and Two Penn Plaza, New York, NY 10121-2289, USA

First published 2008

A catalogue record of this book is available from the British Library

ISBN-13 978 0335 22195 0 (pb)   978 0335 22196 7 (hb)
ISBN-10 0335 22195-5 (pb)   0335 22196-3 (hb)

Library of Congress Cataloging-in-Publication Data
CIP data applied for

Typeset by RefineCatch Limited, Bungay, Suffolk
Printed in the UK by Bell and Bain Ltd, Glasgow.

The *McGraw·Hill* Companies

With thanks to Barbara Bailey for her unstinting patience and administrative support throughout the development of this book.

Contents

List of contributors

The editors

Jackie Kilbane began her career as a learning disability nurse and worked in services for people with a learning disability for many years before moving into organisational and people development roles. Recently she held senior regional and national roles in the NHS in organisational and leadership development.

Jackie has been involved in the evolution & revolution that is person centred planning and thinking, since the early 1980s, after training to become a PATH and MAPs facilitator.

Jackie now works as an Independent Organisation Consultant and facilitator. Person centred thinking, action learning principles, psychodynamic approaches and systemic practice inform this work. She has an M.A. (Econ) in Applied Social Research and an M.A. in Consulting to Organisations from the Tavistock Institute.

Helen Sanderson leads HSA, a development agency exploring how person centred thinking and planning can change people's lives, organisations and communities. She is the expert advisor on person centred planning to the Valuing People Support Team. Helen's PhD is in person centred planning and change, and she is the author of several books, and the co-author of the Department of Health's guidance. Helen also works as part of IAS, a service provider in Greater Manchester. Helen facilitates a circle of support and is a member of Trust Circles North West.

Jeanette Thompson is self-directed support programme manager for Sheffield City Council. She has worked in both the NHS, the university sector and social care. She has edited a number of books on a range of subjects and is passionate about the values and beliefs implicit within person centred planning and self-directed support.

Other contributors

Jonathon Bassett is a trainer for the North West Listen to Me Group. He presents at international and national conferences, facilitates design days, and teaches person centred awareness and person centred thinking. Jonathon says, 'The Person Centred Planning helped my Mum and Nan who were worried about me travelling on the train. After my Person Centred Planning review we looked at what was working and not working and we talked it over. Now they are OK about it. I also got my walking boots.' Jonathon co-wrote *The Best of Both Voices: Person Centred Thinking and Advocacy* with Julie Lunt.

Janet Cobb has a nursing background and has a particular interest in health care in relation to both adults and children with learning disabilities. She worked in the NHS for many years either in clinical or management posts before leaving to join the North West Training and Development Team in 1999 to take up a development post leading on health and learning disability issues across the north-west. Subsequently Janet has developed a number of UK-wide networks with a focus on health issues and people with learning disabilities, and now works freelance.

Barbara Coles is a skilled person centred planning facilitator and trainer. She is a director of Families Leading Planning UK. She is a member of Council for the British Institute for Learning Disabilities and advises the chair on family issues. She is a member of In Control's 'Workforce Intelligence Group' as well as the National and South East regional Workforce Development Teams. She is the Regional co-ordinator for the National Brokerage Network for the Midlands. She provides training and facilitation to families living in Oxford-shire via Oxfordshire Family Support Network. Barbara directly manages her son's support arrangements funded by Direct Payments. She was a co-author of the 'Family Guidance' self audit Checklist for Partnership Boards: 'Families Leading Planning; How are we doing? Where are we going?' launched by the Valuing People Support Team.

Simon Duffy is the Chief Executive of in Control, a national programme to transform the organisation of social care into a system of self-directed support. He has set up several person centred services, such as Inclusion Glasgow, to provide individual support. He has a PhD in Moral Philosophy and is the author of *Keys to Citizenship*.

Liz Evans My name is Liz Evans and I live in the community of Macclesfield in my own home. I have lived here for 20 years. I have a part time job as a volunteer at the local Community Day Service. I am involved in a self advo-cacy group called "Speaking Up and Speaking Out" and I support adults with learning disabilities to learn about speaking up for themselves. I am learning to use British Sign Language and it helps me with the self advocacy work and being a trainer for Person Centred Planning on the awareness days and on the

'Listen to Me' course. I am also the focus person on day 3 of the 'Essential Lifestyle Planning' course.

In my spare time I enjoy swimming, cooking, going to church and going to the theatre in Manchester.

Jo Harvey is a partner in Helen Sanderson Associates, a development agency, the aim of which is to create person centred change. Jo works with organisations to support the development and implementation of person centred services. Currently she leads HSA on support planning and was previously the organisation's lead on person centred teams. Previously, Jo worked for the NHS, both as a senior manager and as a community learning disability nurse.

Chris Hatton has been involved in research with people with learning disabilities for over 15 years. He is Professor of Psychology, Health and Social Care at the Institute for Health Research, Lancaster University, UK, and previously worked as a researcher for many years at the Hester Adrian Research Centre, Manchester University, UK. He has jointly edited or written several books and good practice guides, and over 120 articles in academic and professional journals.

Leah Jones has worked for the Halton Speak Out group for four years, helping people speak up for themselves and be in control of their own lives. Leah's work extends to working in schools with young people in transition, and she has also been involved in training staff in social care and health.

Linda Jordan is the London Regional Advisor for the Valuing People Support Team. Before taking up this position, Linda was Head of Special Educational Needs in the London Borough of Hackney. Linda was previously a teacher and from 1986 to 1994 also an elected councilor in the London Borough of Newham. She is the parent of a young woman with a learning disability.

Jo Kennedy is an independent consultant with a background in community development and community care. She is particularly interested in how community development approaches can be used to support people with learning disabilities or mental health issues with the aim of including them in their communities. Jo has co-written articles for the Joseph Rowntree Foundation and the *Community Development* journal on the contribution community development could make to including people with disabilities. She is also the co-author of two books: *People, Plans and Possibilities: Exploring Person Centred Planning* (SHS 1999) and *Friendship and Community: Practical Suggestions for Making Connections in Community* (NWTDT 2002).

Nizakat Khan works for Oldham Metropolitan Borough Council.

Julie Lunt is a training and development consultant with the development agency Helen Sanderson Associates, where she leads on mental health and is developing work in person centred outcomes. She worked for many years as an Occupational Therapist in the Health Service and was formerly a training associate for BILD. She was a citizen's advocate for 10 years and co-founded a self-advocacy speaking-up group. She says, 'I am using person centred thinking more and more in all aspects of my work. The tools are so effective in helping us to understand the people we support, so that they can get the lives they want. They have also helped me think about my own dreams and aspirations which led me to becoming a full-time consultant. We also use them as a team to help us to work better together and understand how we work individually.' Julie co-wrote *The Best of Both Voices: Person Centred Thinking and Advocacy* with Jonathon Bassett.

Tom McLean is a former NHS Director at the forefront of the hospital closure programme in the north-west of England and has remained interested in the development of alternative and inclusive support systems for people with learning disabilities. This includes the use of direct payments for people with severe learning difficulties through independent living trusts. He is disappointed in some trends which are seeking to congregate larger numbers of people together, in spite of the lessons learned many years ago. He feels that the experiences of the institutions should not be forgotten by the newer generations of commissioners and policy-makers.

Nji Oranu is a qualified social worker registered with the General Social Care Council, who qualified in 2003 from Goldsmiths College, London. Nji has been working in the social care field for over 10 years with particular experience and interest in working with people who have a learning disability or a profound multiple disability from BME backgrounds in inner city boroughs. Previously Nji was a person centred planning co-ordinator and is now a senior practitioner with the 16+ age group leaving care services in Hackney.

Carl Poll is Director of Communications for in Control, the partnership that is playing a key role in the creation of a new system of social care – self-directed support. In 1990, he started KeyRing Living Support Networks, an innovative supported living organisation, which he ran until 2003. In recent years, Carl has contributed to raising a national debate on the meaning of citizenship for marginalised people, for example, organising seminal conferences with speakers such as John McKnight from Chicago and Varun Vidyarthi from Lucknow.

Chris Sholl has over 25 years experience of working with disabled people and their families in a range of settings. Chris was the project director of the West Midlands Transition Pathway Project which produced the Transition Pathway guidance and tools to support person centred transition planning. These are now being used on a national basis and were runner-up for the 'Books for Teaching and Learning Award' 2006, see www.transitionpathway.co.uk. Chris is passionate about improving transition planning in order that young people can lead the adult lives they hope and dream for.

Alison Short is a skilled person centred planning facilitator and trainer, and works extensively with Helen Sanderson Associates, National Development Team and Families Leading Planning U.K. She was the lead author of *Families Leading Planning: A Resource Pack to Enable Families to Take the Lead in Person Centred Planning with and for People with Disabilities that They Love*. Her knowledge of individual budgets and brokerage is also extensive: she works as a broker, has acted as a consultant and trainer with the Life Planning projects, was national lead on support brokerage for the in Control programme, and is now regional co-ordinator for the National Brokerage Network for the south-west.

Louise Skelhorn is a consultant, trainer and mentor who works as a core team member of Helen Sanderson Associates and is part of the Essential Lifestyle Planning Learning Community. Her greatest passion is working with people with the labels of profound and multiple disabilities and communication impairments. She has done so for the past 14 years, integrating total communication techniques within person centred thinking and planning. Louise's professional background was as a learning disability nurse, social worker, person centred planning co-ordinator in human services and she now provides university seminars to student health and social care professionals. Louise has co-authored several books, while continuing her journey of lifelong learning, alongside individuals, families, teams and organisations.

Sam Smith set up and is Executive Director of C-Change for Inclusion, a supported living organisation providing self-directed support to adults with learning difficulties and mental health issues within the Glasgow area. Sam was a former commissioner with the learning disability partnership. She is currently undertaking a PhD exploring perceptions of risk and challenging behaviour.

Michael Smull is the Chair of The Learning Community for Person Centred Approaches and Director of Support Development Associates. He is the co-developer of essential lifestyle planning and has been working with people with disabilities for the past 35 years. He works with government and private agencies to support self-determination and has written extensively on these issues.

Lynne Westwood is a well respected lecturer at the University of Wolver-hampton. As well as delivering support to students to equip them to work in innovative ways in the future, Lynne has a range of research interests that include sensory environments and their value to people who have a learning disability, supporting people who have a profound and multiple learning disability and aromatherapy with people who have a learning disability.

Kim Williams is a speech and language therapist and an associate with Helen Sanderson Associates. Kim specialises in working with people with the label learning disability and has done so for the past 19 years, within the arena of health care. Kim is committed to the development of best practice regarding the integration of total communication techniques within person centred thinking and planning. Kim's interests lie in the creation of bespoke training packages and resources to empower others to create an environment that supports positive change and communicative interactions, within an individual's experience.

Introduction

Jeanette Thompson, Jackie Kilbane and Helen Sanderson

Writing and editing this book has been a journey that has taken place at a time of significant change in health and social care. While this book was in the process of being written, self-directed support has become common language for many people. This has built on the visions created in the development of person centred planning and within the independent living movement. Those advocating a self-directed support approach find themselves actively searching for answers to the following questions:

1   How does citizenship work in my life – in terms of direction, money, home, support, ability to have control over important things and a life within my community?
2   To what degree do these issues operate in the lives of people who have a learning disability and have they been able to achieve better lives and citizenship?
3   What factors prevent the person who has a learning disability from being a citizen and how can these be overcome?

These are questions that have actively occupied those of us who have edited this text; they have formed a key part of our professional background (which for each of us started in the NHS) and our development as professionals working with people who have a learning disability. During the time we have been editing this book, interest has also grown in relation to the ways in which self-directed support can work within a health-care context, with some places integrating continuing health-care monies within individual budgets.

As well as working with the challenges of a new way of delivering services that put people more in control of their lives, the structures or ways of working with people have also developed. We have moved from our collective and individual positions of trying to understand how to help people find better lives and be listened to, by using approaches such as person centred planning, to one where we are now starting to understand and define person centred practice and all its constituent parts.

Important within this journey of self-directed support and person centred practice is the position of health and social care services and the contribution of health and social care professionals. This book clearly articulates the many ways in which professionals can participate within the person centred practice agenda and subsequently develop the self-directed support approach to aid people who have a learning disability.

This is discussed in the context of person centred practice and its evolution, key partnerships and the way in which these contribute to the current agenda, the strategies to meet the needs of people with a learning disability and a focus on the future, and how to consolidate person centred practice in all that we do.

This book includes chapters that focus upon the historical development of person centred practice, the development of a model to inform person centred practice for use by professionals and the tools and skills to inform that role. This book identifies that the key partnership that needs to be supported is the one with people who have a learning disability and this is developed in the chapters that consider how these partnerships can be extended to health and professional education. Chapters 6–9 explore the needs of different groups of people, including those with communication needs, people from different cultural backgrounds and those young people moving into adulthood. Finally, Chapters 10–13 look at people who have a learning disability making their own plans, with Families Leading Planning, and how we are able to move towards person centred approaches to support planning and greater community inclusion.

When professionals integrate these concepts and approaches into their day-to-day work, we believe we will have moved from placing people at the centre of our interventions to understanding where we fit in the context of the person and their control over their own life. We will also have moved from working to implement person centred plans to creating a culture of person centred practice that enables the full participation of people with disabilities as citizens with all that this encompasses.

1 Exploring the history of person centred practice

Jackie Kilbane with Tom McLean

Key issues

- Historical overview of learning disability services
- History of person centred planning and thinking
- Historical context for professional involvement in planning with people

Introduction

This chapter explores the historical context for person centred thinking and planning, and the involvement of professionals in planning. This will locate person centred planning within both a historical and an organisational context. The chapter sets the scene for the use of person centred thinking, planning and the positive support strategies of professionals as we move towards more person centred practice. This analysis is intended to encourage professionals to think about the way that the environment in which they operate can both support and challenge person centredness. It is not the intention to offer an exhaustive, detailed history, but more usefully to summarise and offer aspects of the history that inform practices and experiences as we move into new professional work futures and as people with learning disabilities and their families move into whole life futures.

This chapter will therefore briefly consider the history of learning disability services, outlining the gradual journey that includes the development of work practices that are increasingly focused upon the experience and expertise of the person receiving support. We explore person centred planning and thinking as an integral part of supporting a person to plan, organise their life, and experience citizenship. We examine the importance of people who have a learning disability taking control back from external agencies and how we meet the challenges to implement and embed person centred practice.

In order to achieve this, the chapter is organised into three sections:

1   an historical organisational context of learning disability services;
2   the development of person centred planning: evolution and revolution;
3   professional involvement in people's plans and planning.

However, before embarking on the main body of this chapter we wish to deal with two points. The first relates to the authors' professional backgrounds, as we are both learning disability nurses, albeit from different generations! This is relevant in that we will use personal practice flashbacks to illustrate and highlight historical issues and experiences throughout the chapter. Most of our flashbacks and stories are drawn from our experiences as nurses in different settings. Through these, we offer detail on the historical workings of professional power within large institutions during the long and winding road towards the final closure of large, segregated environments, a road that has, at the time of publication, still to end for a number of people in the UK. This emphasis is both a strength and a weakness of the chapter. However, we make no apology for sharing our uniquely located experiences to explore the history of learning disability services and planning with people. As you, the reader, follow this exploration of the history of learning disability services and person centred planning, we invite you to consider what is shared and what is different between what we describe and your own experiences from your unique background, current practice and professional identity.

The second point to note is the place of people who have a learning disability within the stories that we tell. No one is better placed to tell these stories than people with learning disabilities themselves. What they tell us about their experiences of support services past and present is often powerful and moving as well as offering us a valuable window into lived experiences of surviving institutions and services. As there is insufficient space here to do some of these individual stories justice, readers are directed to the annotated bibliography at the end of this chapter as a source of recommended and valuable further reading by people who have lived institutional and community lives.

An historical organisational context of learning disability services

A century of institutionalisation

We only really began to hear about any kind of organised services for people during the Industrial Revolution at the turn of the twentieth century. There were institutions before then, though these were usually established as a result of charitable donations, for example, the Royal Albert Hospital in Lancaster opened in 1870, this later became part of the newly created NHS in 1948 (CSV 2006). As the Industrial Revolution began to develop, more people moved to cities, community lives changed and people became more valuable for the perceived quantity and quality of their contribution to society. The differences of people with learning disabilities in relation to others in society were apparent and they were subsequently identified as defective. However, there was at this time also a relatively benevolent (compared to what followed) pattern of 'care and education' established within these early institutions. This tentative hope in individuals and in the practice of education for people seen to be different from others was overtaken at the start of the twentieth century when academic leaders of that time identified people with learning disabilities as both an actual and potential drain upon societal productiveness and as a risk to the quality of an idealised 'race' (Race 1994). This change in attitude heralded the eugenics movement (Tredgold 1909), where people with learning disabilities were the focus of segregation and control. This resulted in people with learning disabilities being moved into large institutions away from highly populated areas. Eugenics is the practice of 'race improvement', informing not only segregation of the sexes and sterilisation of women but also encompassing the atrocities of Nazi Germany during the Second World War.

The 1913 Mental Deficiency Act (HMSO 1913), the 1959 Mental Health Act (HMSO 1959) and the introduction of the National Health Service in 1946 (HMSO 1946) were all important in ensuring the rise of the hospital institution. This was reflected in the increasing numbers of people classed as 'mentally deficient' and those who were required to live in hospital institutions. In addition, this period of history saw the dominance of the medical model of care. Consequently, developments during this time typically involved the classification of the disabilities of people living within institutions (Box 1.1).

Care and caring practices in institutions continued to consistently classify people with learning disabilities as significantly less valuable than others up until the mid-1900s. At that time, research findings began to backtrack and there was some optimism about what was seen to be a small potential for work and employment. Links were beginning to be made between the quality of the environment and the quality of work contributed by people. In addition, there was then the beginning of a growing understanding that institutional life was permanent for most people and living conditions there were very poor.

Institutional life was medicalised, with rigid hierarchies. Men and women lived separately under the naïve assumption from those in positions of power that this would mean an absence of sexual activity. Classifications of people's ability were used to allocate jobs and those seen to be most able were often used to provide care for those people who were seen to be less able, blurring the boundaries between patient and worker (Mitchell 2000).

Box 1.1 Practice flashback: early professional role

Case notes from the early twentieth century show that the professional role was that of the mental welfare officer, who was responsible for managing the boundaries of entry into institutions at that time. When welfare officers first became involved in the lives of people with a disability, decisions were made about 'disposal'. The availability of a bed in an institution would be followed by an assessment of abilities, usually by a psychiatrist and later by a psychologist, and later still by multidisciplinary teams as they came on board in the late 1960s. These assessments led to decisions, more about service arrangements and fitting people in, than personal wishes, for example, in hospitals a person with epilepsy would be allocated a bed in an 'EP' (epilepsy) ward, irrespective of any other consideration.

Back to the future: institution to community

In the latter half of the 1900s, there were again significant developments in thinking, practice and policy that formed and reshaped services for people with learning disabilities. There was debate during the last half of the century about where and how people with learning disabilities should be cared for; whether to locate them within mental health services within the local authority or within emerging health services. Social care was identified and defined in the late 1960s with the formation of social services. There were efforts to improve conditions in learning disability hospitals that gathered momentum following the publication of reports, such as the Report of the Howe Committee into events at Ely Hospital in 1969 (HMSO 1969), that were highly critical of conditions and emphasised the seriousness of problems within long-stay hospital institutions. Policy development following this included the 1971 White Paper *Better Services for the Mentally Handicapped* (Dept of Health 1971). This White Paper targeted shifting the balance of care settings from hospital to community, noting deficiencies in the current system and identifying models for daytime activity.

Alongside these policy developments ideas and theories emerged that were equally significant. Early in this phase was the significant influence of normalisation. Wolfensberger (1972) gave substance to the concept and development of normalisation by formulating a method of service evaluation called PASS (Programme Analysis of Service Systems), using principles of normalisation; although the normalisation concept was being developed overseas during the 1960s, it was not until the mid-1970s that its impact was felt in the UK and during the 1970s and 1980s PASS and its successor PASSING were a powerful though contested instrument of change. The principles of normalisation were used to develop 'service accomplishments' (O'Brien and Tyne 1981): community presence, choice (Box 1.2), competence, respect and community participation and these were generally better known in UK services than normalisation. Local plans were drawn up to develop ideas about community-based services. One of the most highly regarded of these was *A Model District Service* (RHA 1983), that again drew upon the principles of normalisation.

Other factors that influenced the phase of system reform and led to change include the growth of the human rights and civil rights movements, promoting social justice, and the development of theory relating to groups of people at risk of devaluation and marginalisation (Bradley 2005). Theories about models of disability impacted upon thinking and practice at the time, including the social model of disability which challenged the medicalised identification of disability as a condition and offered critical thinking about the ways that disability is constructed in our social world. The Inclusion Movement (leaders of inclusion were Judith Snow, Marsha Forest, John O'Brien and Jack Pearpoint (O'Brien and O'Brien 2001)) emphasised the rights of people to participate in communities and to have opportunities in mainstream and non-segregated settings, challenging unhelpful assumptions about the abilities of people (disabled and non-disabled) to connect with and live alongside each other.

Key legislative developments that were important influencers of service development included the Jay Report (HMSO 1979). This looked into the care of people with a learning disability and the training of staff. It was the training recommendations, not at all liked by those with vested interests, which led to it being largely shelved. However, the chapters on ordinary housing, the inclusion of people, and support, based upon the needs and wishes of individuals, were influential over the next few years. This gave support to the integration of people into the life of the community (Box 1.3), contributing to the radical rethink about how care was organised and delivered. In addition, in

---

Box 1.2 Practice flashback: choice

The concept of the five service accomplishments did much to educate staff about what was possible, about how to improve people's lives and accord respect and dignity to individuals by thinking about the exercise of choice by people with a learning disability, including those who do not communicate using words. The learning extended from simple choice issues such as food and clothing preferences to the development of much more imaginative ways of getting to know people well and identifying what people might like in their whole lives and futures.

Box 1.3 Practice flashback: experiences of resettlement

The closures of large hospitals were greeted with different responses, depending on where you were in that system. People with learning disabilities, families, professionals and care staff had very different experiences. For some people with learning disabilities, a move out of a large congregate setting meant confusing disruption to routines held for decades and enforced separation from friends and companions. For others, leaving the hospital meant a transition into a more peaceful, varied and dignified phase of life, living with just a few other people and supported by people whom one had known for years. Family members received calls from resettlement workers as the shift to community care began; family members were asked to consider having relatives live with them after years of separation and some families misunderstood, thinking that this would be the only option – it was not clear, at least at first, that provision could take a number of forms. Other family members who had visited relatives in hospital institutions worked hard to try to ensure that the person was safe and secure in any new place they were to live. People who worked in institutions braced themselves for change; nurses moved from running a ward full of people requiring physical care to being a manager of three supported tenancies with individual staff teams. Care staff went from helping ten people have a bath before 9am to helping two people get ready to go to a day centre. People living all over the UK began to experience neighbours with learning disabilities for the first time, some were welcoming and others not.

1980, the Kings Fund developed the 'Ordinary Life' series that advocated the shift towards residential care and an emphasis on ordinary housing. The 1990 NHS and Community Care Act sealed the legislative developments that shaped the new era of community.

These disparate strands of experience, depending upon your position in the system of hospitals, care and the community, reflect how problematic it is when we try to offer a simple, single history of support for people with learning disabilities. Often it is easier now to think generally about the 'old institutions' and the history of government policy and resulting shifts in models of service provision, rather than explore the parallel processes that we all go through: as patients at the time, workers, family members, neighbours, as people, in order to make and accommodate changes in response to the situations we are faced with.

The values and attitudes that had first led to the mass segregation of people with learning disabilities were now leading us towards new patterns of services. We began to hear and learn more about empowerment of people with disabilities advocacy and the 'quality of life' debate, which again reflected shifting attitudes towards those people. Community services were usually organised into a few fields: residential care in the form of group homes; day services in segregate, congregate settings; some college courses; short breaks services; and community teams that employed a number of different professionals including learning disability nurses, social workers (later care managers), occupational therapists and psychologists.

The twenty-first-century citizen

We have chosen not to offer a practice flashback in this section about the start of the twenty-first century, as this is not yet 'history'! We do, however, offer space at the end of the section as a reader exercise to create your own practice snapshot.

The White Paper, *Valuing People: A New Strategy for Learning Disability for the 21st Century* (Department of Health 2001) in England, *The Same As You?* (SE 2000) in Scotland and *Fulfilling the Promises* (WAG 2001) in Wales have been recent and significant policy developments in the UK. In *Valuing People*, four key principles of rights, independence, choice and inclusion underpinned ambitious proposals for changing services and lives for the better. Person centred planning was seen as a significant approach that would be a key tool in making these cultural changes (Routledge et al. 2002).

It is possible to make clear connections between service developments in the last half of the twentieth century and the principles embedded in *Valuing People*. For example, the emphasis on Inclusion reflects a passion for social inclusion and being with. The emphasis on rights is grounded in legislation such as the Human Rights Act 1998 and the Disability Discrimination Act 1995.

Two themes have emerged through policy, practice, service and conceptual developments in the past few decades that are important now in the development of services. These are the linked concepts of *individualisation/personalisation* and *choice/control*.

The emphasis upon individualisation or personalisation and increasing choices is unsurprising in learning disability services, given the dissatisfaction with mass segregation and congregation that dominated the last century. The themes of personalisation and choice are also evident in wider policy development. For example, the White Paper, *Our Health, Our Care, Our Say* (Department of Health 2006) includes goals of 'choice and a louder voice'. A number of ways to put more control in the hands of the person requiring support have emerged in the past ten years, including the use of independent living funds and direct payments.

In the development of person centred planning, Smull (2001) identified a useful way to think about choice in the lives of people with learning disabilities. These ideas help us to think about the complexity of choosing, at a time when choice is given a lot of emphasis in government policy. Choice is made up of interdependent aspects that all need to be present for us to make a choice:

- preferences – knowing what you want;
- opportunity – to do what you want;
- control – the authority to satisfy a preference.

In recent times, there has been a move towards a clearer separation of the person from the traditional service, through the development of self-directed support. If *Valuing People* has set out an agenda for what needs to be done, self-directed support is, for many people, a way to achieve the vision in *Valuing People*, whether this is through receiving direct payments or another form of individualised funding. Wolfensberger (1972) noted the 'extraordinary control' over people as a result of the mass segregation of people with learning disabilities and though service structures are now changing, control over people is proving trickier to dispense with. Self-directed support has significant potential to increase the choices people make about their support and the control they have over that support.

Another concept that is important in current society and in the development of learning disability services that is congruent with the shift towards personalisation and choice is citizenship. Duffy (2003) offers six keys to citizenship that reflect the principles of *Valuing People*, where possessing the six keys enables individuals to achieve citizenship. Supporting people to move towards and achieve citizenship is one of the central challenges facing us over the next few years. The six keys are:

1   Self-determination – the authority to control our own lives.
2   Direction – a plan or idea of what we want to achieve.
3   Money – to live and to control our own life.
4   Home – a place that is our own and a base for life.
5   Support – help to do things we need help to achieve.
6   Community life – an active engagement in the life of the community and the development of our own network of relationships.

Making choices is central to people with learning disabilities being full citizens, making choices about support, money, direction and community life. Citizenship and the applications of person centred planning offer us a framework to support people to make choices that make it more likely that they will have good support services.

For the first time, the implementation of a model for self-directed support and citizenship is targeted not only at people with learning disabilities, but also at other groups of people who receive services, for example, older people and disabled people. We will need to wait some time, however, before we can consider from a historical perspective what these recent developments mean in terms of better lives for people.

Activity 1.1

From institutional life to community life to my life

Think about someone you know who has spent a significant portion of her/his life in learning disability institutions and who is still supported by services in some way today. Recount their story here using a life timeline – focus on life-changing events to shape the timeline.

Sample timeline: Ewan
Born 1934 . . . 1947 moved to Ollerton House . . . 1967 moved wards due to poor behaviour . . . 1984 moved to group home . . . 1994 married Jane . . . 2000 moved into a flat with Jane.
For the same person, think about and list the differences between their institutional life, their life in the community and their life right now, wherever that is. Consider each of the following areas: who they live with, how much money is available to them, how they spend their time, who supports them, and what has changed over time?
Now use this information to develop your own Practice Flashback, taking particular note of the factors that are influencing you as a practitioner right now, both professionally and organisationally. In your Practice Flashback you may also want to consider which of these influences helps and hinders the people you support to be active citizens. Duffy's six keys to citizenship could be a useful framework for this.

What the histories of learning disability services show is that current societal attitudes regarding groups of people significantly impact upon the way these groups of people are treated; there is a mirroring of the history of societal views and attitudes towards people with learning disabilities and the way they have been treated. The historical organisational context of learning disability is entwined with the practices and ways of working that reflect policy shifts and our changing attitudes. As we move now into the era of explicitly valuing people, safeguarding the choices and rights of people with learning disabilities and giving them good support as citizens, we have a parallel movement of citizenship and person centred practice that offers ways of working that embody and reflect these attitudes. We are in a unique position whereby some of the value-driven movements and the policy context have dovetailed. This has been guided by the efforts of opinion leaders who have made inroads into the central political decision-making structures in the UK and through the continued hard work of people working in and on the edges of organisations that shape the present and future of how we work with people with learning disabilities. This, of course, has created different tensions between the different groups of people who all have a stake in the development of services and support for people with learning disabilities.

The next section takes a closer look at the development of person centred planning and thinking and the ways this can help resolve some of these tensions.

The development of person centred planning: evolution and revolution

The title of this section is deliberate in that it moves away from a binary notion of the development of person centred planning. The emergence of person centred planning is not a simple case of evolution *or* revolution. The development of person centred planning contains elements of both evolution *and* revolution. Some evolutionary elements of person centred planning can be traced back through historical development of services and other elements have made conceptual leaps in understanding the empowerment of people through planning. Person centred planning emerged in the UK through the work of practitioners who 'held a line' on embodying a set of clear, explicit values and principles throughout a process of planning that includes the individual making desired changes to their lives.

In the UK, planning in the institutional days was limited, it was only with the beginning of the shift away from hospital institutions that practices concerning plans and planning also shifted. In the institution the power of decision-making was clearly with the professional, and decisions about what was *important for* people, rather than *important to* people, were dominant (Box 1.4).

While the practice flashback clearly demonstrates elements of *important for* aspects of working with people, *important to* is necessary if we are to move towards the goal of citizenship. Important to/for has developed as a key person centred thinking skill (see Chapters 3 and 11 for more detailed information) that can be used to increase the focus on what is important to people and to work creatively with what is seen to be important for a person. Another tool, the 'doughnut' (detailed in Chapter 3) can be used by professionals as it looks at 'roles' in helping people to have what is important to and for them.

One of the first mentions of plans in policy documents as an aspect of support for people with a learning disability came in the Jay Report (HMSO 1979); the concept of a life plan was introduced as a way of identifying the needs of people with learning disabilities and achieving co-ordination across

Box 1.4 Practice flashback: making plans

The case notes or file and simple employment and activity records comprised the plan, the only planning for the people concerned in institutions. People themselves would talk endlessly about wanting to get out of the place, go to another ward, have boy or girl friends, get married, have visits, and go home. Whether these dreams, desires and wishes were taken into account is another issue ... Indeed, whether wants, as opposed to professionally identified needs ever came into the process is questionable. Perhaps, in terms of spending small amounts of money, going on a trip or not going (certainly not choosing the actual destination), choosing, in other words, from a small number of options did begin to grow with the adoption of less restrictive regimes.

The 'card' listed daily activities, whether this was work in a hospital department, such as the farm, sewing room, laundry ward-based cleaning or kitchen work, or attending a department to do craft work or make artefacts for use in the hospital or for sale – brushes, shoes, for example. Similar records would show a timetable for domestic and social activity such as walks, dances, haircuts and bathing. Changes to personal routines would follow a discussion between the charge nurse and the doctor on his rounds. The 'patient' would usually be present, being kept back from work to be placed 'in front of the doctor'. This presence was, often, the total extent of personal involvement; the patient may or may not have been included in the discussions and decisions which could lead to a change of ward, of work or activity.

A more open case-conference approach to larger decisions in the life of patients was established as more people became aware of and took up more modern practices. Therapy, training or workplace staff would be consulted; this approach could be subverted by 'emergency or urgent' decisions being taken by the doctor on the daily round. The need to find a suitable vacancy for a new admission could lead to five or six chequerboard-style ward-to-ward moves for people. Case conferences were often used for purposes other than to advance the care and support and development of the person concerned – demonstration of conditions and syndromes, for example. This could be confusing and even more so when the same meeting was used for more than one purpose. Frustration with a medically dominated system was evident in the late 1960s as extensions of case conferences began to take on the views of more professional groups and become more developmental rather than treatment-focused in their approaches. These meetings provided the base from which the multidisciplinary approach developed.

services. The origins of planning with people include Individual Programme Plans (IPPs) (Box 1.5) or Individual Planning (IPs). This key practice development reflected the prominence of individualisation during the 1970s, the 1980s and the 1990s. It was a significant development in that it applied principles of individualisation of plans and involved the person with a learning disability in decision-making. A positive, though undeveloped progression from IPPs was Shared Action Planning (SAP). Advocated by the Open University, this approach increased the element of partnership in the development of action plans.

Sanderson et al. (1997) summarise a number of concepts and practices that form the origins of person centred planning that have already been explored within the previous section. These are:

- normalisation
- the social model of disability and the disability movement
- the five accomplishments
- institutional closure
- the Inclusion Movement
- dissatisfaction with Individual Planning
- best practice in social work assessment.

In North America where person centred planning originated, there was a community of practice approach to the development of person centred planning which took place between 1979 and 1992, O'Brien and O'Brien (2002) refer to this as the 'formative years' of person centred planning. The term 'community of practice' was used, as there were a number of people interested in person centred planning who were prepared not only to share and learn both knowledge and skills, but also to offer one another peer support. Some people involved in the community of practice were informed

---

Box 1.5 Practice flashback: IPPs

Large groups of professionals met to examine strengths and weaknesses (later described as needs), decide priorities, set goals, design and refine programmes which, when implemented by therapy, care or nursing staff, would deliver progress for the person concerned. People could emerge from IPP meetings with 15 goals, ranging from tying shoelaces to managing money to resolving incontinence, and mostly seen as addressing their identified weaknesses. The sheer quantity of goals could be daunting and could result in them being put in the drawer till the next review. Often plans of this kind achieved a more purposeful use of time for people, and had a positive connection with perceptions of personal need and for those reasons were an improvement on former practices.

by the principles of normalisation in developing services. Leading figures in the formative phase who were developing person centred planning styles, began to teach and run workshops in the UK where distinctive planning styles that had been developed in the US were introduced.

In the past 20 years, four styles of person centred planning have become available and used here in the UK:

- *Personal Futures Planning* (Mount 1987) is a planning process that involves getting to know the person and what life is like now, developing ideas about what he or she would like in the future and taking action to move towards this. It involves exploring possibilities within the community and looking at what needs to change within services. The process is colourfully recorded in words and pictures using different 'maps'. This planning style draws upon the five service accomplishments.

- *Essential Lifestyle Planning* (Smull and Harrison 1992) was developed to enable people to move out of long-stay institutions. It is a way to learn who and what is important to people in their day-to-day lives and how to support them to have the lifestyle that they want, while staying healthy and safe.

- *MAPs* (Vandercook, York and Forest 1989) have a section at the beginning of the process to record the history of a person. MAPs ask the questions, 'Who is the person?' and 'What are his or her gifts?' People express hopes and fears for the future as part of the process. The action plan then becomes about moving towards hopes and dreams and moving away from nightmares and fears. This is a planning style that was introduced as part of the Inclusion Movement.

- *PATH* (Pearpoint, O'Brien and Forest 1993) can be used as a planning style with individuals and with organisations. It helps people with a basic commitment to the person to sharpen their sense of a desirable future and to plan how to make progress. It assumes that those present know and care about the individual and are committed to supporting the person to attain a desirable future. PATH is not about gathering information about a person but is a way of planning direct and immediate action. This is also a planning style that was introduced as part of the Inclusion Movement.

It was with the arrival of person centred planning that we really began to get serious about trying to consider and then follow up someone's wishes and preferences. Up until this point, planning in the traditional sense had primarily been about (1) how to make a government-driven change to services; and (2) how to make a professionally judged change.

In the UK, person centred planning is unusual in that an emergent set of practices has become embedded within policy development and implementation, as we saw in the presence of person centred planning in *Valuing People* and the subsequent implementation guidance for Partnership Boards (Department of Health 2002). Since 2002, many people have developed some sort of person centred plan and we have learned much about what it takes to make a positive difference to a person's life through the process of planning and implementing plans. During this time, there have been developments in person centred planning and some of these are described here:

- *person centred thinking*: person centred thinking uses tools that are discrete building blocks of person centred planning. These tools began to be used on their own, as ways to change practice on a daily basis. This book explores how these tools can be used by professionals, specifically in Chapters 3, 7 and 11.
- *person centred planning applications*: in practice, there are several points in a person's life when person centred planning and thinking can be applied to inform and shape how they can live and consequently how professionals support them. Some of these are the focus of chapters in this book and include significant life transitions, addressing and managing health issues, and support planning.

The next section explores issues relating to professional involvement in people's plans and planning, in light of the development of person centred planning and thinking and shifts in the ways that services are provided.

Professional involvement in people's plans and planning

Shared space, shared story?

Professionals are people who have qualifications and experience in their chosen field of work and are paid to provide a service to people, based upon what they know. The history of people with learning disabilities has long been intertwined with the histories of institutions and those who choose to work within them. By institution, we refer not only to large, isolated institutional buildings where many people with learning disabilities have spent their lives during the last century (and some still do), but also to the plethora of human services that includes group homes, supported tenancies, day centres and hospitals. Individual professionals and professional groups working within public, private and not-for-profit organisations have a stake in the well-being and quality of life of people with learning disabilities. Mitchell (2000) has considered to what extent there can be a shared history between people with learning disabilities and those who work with them. His work suggests that the historical boundaries between hospital, institution, resident and worker have sometimes been ambiguous, for example, work tasks were similar but the pay received for work was different. Historically, the institutional space was shared, but the stories were not. The distinction between a shared space and shared story is important. The partialness of what is shared highlights what can be a gulf between people with learning disabilities and the professionals who become involved in their lives.

Activity 1.2

Reflecting on your role with people who have a learning disability, how different is your understanding of the experience of what you offer the person to their lived experience? How much do you gain from the continued dependence on the current structures that place people who have a learning disability? What can you do to change this?

A lot has been written about the dependence of people with learning disabilities on the services that support them. However, highlighted here is the partial dependence of professionals upon people with learning disabilities for their learning and successful working lives. As professionals employed to work with people with learning disabilities, there is a risk that we are already implicated in the maintenance of dependence and location of learning disabled people as less valuable than others in society in some way, widening the gap between the enablers and the enabled. Many professionals have benefited from the constancy of learning disabled people's support requirements and their long struggle for more independence, because it has meant we can contribute to people's lives and well-being in our time at work. This location of our professional selves as interdependent with those we work with in shared spaces can be useful as we move towards sharing power in person centred practice.

Professions have evolved and developed over time. One of the outcomes of deepening professional distinctions over time is an increased clarity about where the boundaries are between the varied contributions of professional groups, alongside a growing evidence basis for many professional interventions and activities. This has the potential to be a positive development for people with learning disabilities, in that people (people with learning disabilities, their families and direct care staff) can be clear about where to go for support with different issues.

Professionals have made significant contributions to the care and support of people in the history of services, and all professions can identify positive improvements to ways of working over time. Each profession will be able to identify a pathway through history that has focused upon changing what we do and how we do it to become more effective in some way. And yet . . . how much have people's lives changed as a result? This is a tough and critical question and the intention here is not to attribute blame; we have already explored some of the interdependent aspects of societal attitudes, the development of learning disability services and planning with people. We think that central to more people gaining the life and support that they want is the journey away from a professional gift model and towards a citizenship model (see Chapter 4 for more details). The essence of this shift is about moving the balance of power and control over the way you live your life and how the support you receive is decided and organised, away from professionals and organisations towards people who require support. The next section explores issues of power between professionals and people requiring support.

What's power got to do with it?

Exploring the history of learning disability services shows us that people with learning disabilities have been segregated, devalued and oppressed as a group in society. People with learning disabilities have not had 'a great deal' in society and time. Their physical space, activities and relationships have often been managed by others. These historical patterns have resulted in the authority of people with learning disabilities being contested, including the power to know, to be expert in one's own life, to record and keep any plans made (Box 1.6).

As we move towards more person centred practice for professionals, we continue to learn about how to make useful and significant contributions to people's lives and support. Kilbane and Thompson (2004) identified four

---

Box 1.6 Practice flashback: making and keeping plans

Leaving larger institutions for smaller-scale life in the community prompted a boom in photography, video and memory books. It is important that this is not lost. Until relatively recently, little was done to compensate people with poor memory. There is an obligation on support systems to make serious attempts to keep plans, records of progress and implementation with reviews and pictures, for the benefit of new supporters and for the persons themselves. The emerging picture of people who use person centred plans is a more holistic one than could ever be derived from reading a case note. Sometimes case notes and clinical or social care records say nothing personal, descriptive, positive or nice about individuals; they record events, problems, incidents – the person is seen only as a bundle of needs and problems.

challenges that person centred planning and thinking can present to professionals:

1 Relinquishing control over what happens in a person's life in order to take up a support role.
2 Professional responsibilities and duty of care.
3 Conflict with 'fix it' thinking.
4 The growing emphasis on natural supports.

Moving towards person centred practice means finding and using practical and positive strategies to enable and support people, using professional experience and expertise. Professionals are challenged to work with people using expertise, without becoming 'the expert', and to know and care about someone's struggle with health or social issues, without becoming a fixer. Meeting these challenges requires professionals to listen carefully to what is important to people at the time of their involvement and to act with careful intent in people's lives, using and sharing professional power to support citizenship.

A framework for professional involvement in people's plans and person centred practice is explored in Chapter 2, while specific strategies and their applications are identified in Chapters 3, 7 and 11.

Professional power and authority come from being part of a large structured profession, having specific knowledge about a subject, from your position in a service hierarchy and through passion for what you do. All professionals need to work within their professional boundaries (even when these are often elastic!) and be involved to a greater or lesser extent in the activities of associated professional agencies. Sometimes, specific ways of working emerge in a profession that are expected to be adopted by everyone using that professional title. An example of this in nursing was the Nursing Process (Box 1.7).

Box 1.7 Practice flashback: the Nursing Process

In the nursing profession, a system known as the Nursing Process emerged in the 1970s. This was single disciplinary and was inflicted upon many nursing services including learning disability services, primarily because nurses were managed at a strategic level by districts which were mostly acute-illness centred. This was a setback for multidisciplinary work, but did not hamper the longer-term emergence of person centred and partnership work. The Nursing Process contained, as do all other systems, similar elements. These are cyclic and contain basic steps: assessment, goal setting, implementation, evaluation and review and return to re-assessment.

What was useful about a process such as this was the staged cycle of thinking about what you do, doing it, seeing how it worked and thinking again about what to do next. This is a reflective cycle that is helpful for people involved in supporting others so that learning through and from experiences is maximised (Schön 1983). Most professionals use some sort of reflective process in their work and the best of these involve the people supported. This is essential to person centred practice and enables learning about how to successfully support people and use your professional expertise effectively and appropriately. Some of the person centred thinking tools that can be used for reflective learning about your role in people's plans and planning include what's working/not working and the 4 plus 1 questions (see Chapter 3).

Navigating organisational life

Professionals often belong to more than one institution such as a professional body or organisation and an employing institution. As a professional you have some accountability to each, in addition, you have accountability to the customer or person you are invited to work with in your professional role. This diffuse accountability can be problematic for the professional moving towards person centred practice (Box 1.8).

This practice flashback is more recent and probably familiar to lots of people reading this book. Professionals employed in services have often told us stories about feeling that they offer a service and support to people *in spite of*

Box 1.8 Practice flashback: an example of surviving institutional change

I had three different service reconfigurations to deal with within two years; this is pretty usual for public services. These restructures were moving from having four geographical community learning disability teams to three teams across the city, integrating Care Managers into what had previously been 'health' teams, shifting from being employed by one PCT (primary care trust) to another and finally, moving offices four times. Each of these changes, big and small were outside of my control and resulted in changes to both the people I supported and the colleagues I worked alongside. Restructuring took up huge amounts of energy and time when I would have preferred to use my energy to make a difference in people's lives; it felt like these precious resources were being syphoned off to accommodate imposed change. I am sure that the changes were necessary for the survival of the service, but there was a clear cost to both workers and people coming into contact with services and these had little to do with the lives of people with learning disabilities.

the structure and culture of the organisations they work in. We would hope that professionals involved in the lives of people with learning disabilities are part of organisations where there is openness, clear accountability and thoughtful application of values, but this is often not the case and we must survive and hopefully thrive in all sorts of complex environments and complicated service structures. Thriving in this context means finding ways to work as individuals, in teams and in organisations so that more people with learning disabilities find places in society as full citizens.

Bridges (2003) writes about change being different from transition, where change is the external process and transition is the internal process of letting go of an existing set of practices and starting to take on new practices. As an evidence base for person centred planning emerges (Robertson et al. 2005), the challenges that person centred planning, thinking and practice present mean that professionals are expected to think about, respond to and reflect upon new ways of working and make transitions from one set of practices to another, informed by person centred principles. Moving towards person centred practice means navigating through imposed change and making the transitions necessary for moving forward.

Conclusion

The historical patterns of organised services for people with learning disabilities, government policy and legislation, underlying societal attitudes to people's differences, the emergence of professional practices and routines and the vested interests of those in positions of power to influence the rhythms and pace of change are interconnected and interdependent. They inform where we are today and where we go from here. We have followed a path from the past into the present so that we might be better able to work with and through this complexity and make our contribution in our professional roles to more people having the life and support they want. Wheatley (2002) suggests that all change starts when people get together and talk about the things they really care about. She states that questions arising from these conversations are the kinds of questions that connect us all as people and professionals.

On this basis, we invite individual professionals, teams of professionals and professional organisations to continue to ask thoughtful questions about their work in relation to person centred planning, thinking and practice, both present and future. In the dialogue between people that can follow thoughtful questions, we may be able to learn more from our past and present about how to work with and alongside people in ways that enhance life experiences and maximise well-being, not on professional terms, but on the terms of those people receiving our support.

Annotated bibliography

Atkinson, D., Nind, M., Rolph, S. and Welshman, J. (2005) *Witnesses to Change: Families, Learning Difficulties and History*. Kidderminster: BILD Publications.
The stories in *Witnesses to Change* show how learning disabilities have impacted on family life and relationships in the twentieth century, how challenges were approached and how families acted as advocates. It illustrates diversity and variety in family life, aiming to be inclusive and to challenge stereotypes. It highlights past mistakes as well as successes in managing learning disability services. And above all, it celebrates the lives of families who have contributed their stories. Annotation taken from the Open University learning disability history health and social care research group. See www.open.ac.uk/hsc/idsite/research.grp for more information.

Bradley, A. (2005) *Understanding Support Services for People with Learning Disabilities*. Kidderminster: BILD Publications.
This is a clear and concisely written workbook about the history of learning disability, the concept of and models of disability, person centred planning and the current context of support services.

CSV (2006) Community Service Volunteers Royal Albert Hospital Archive: Unlocking the Past.
The Royal Albert Hospital has a useful historical archive and resource that traces the history of this north-west England institution: www.unlockingthepast.org.uk

O'Brien, J. and O'Brien, C.L. (2002) *Implementing Person Centered Planning: Voices of Experience*. Toronto: Inclusion Press.
This edited book brings together contributions from people involved in the leadership, development and implementation of person centred planning. Chapters cover lots of diverse aspects of planning with people, including helping staff support choice, defining features of person centred planning and developing facilitators.

Further reading

Atkinson, D., Jackson, M. and Walmsley, J. (1997) *Forgotten Lives: Exploring the History of Learning Disability*. Kidderminster: BILD Publications.
Atkinson, D., McCarthy, M., Walmsley, J. et al. (2000) *Good Times, Bad Times: Women with Learning Difficulties Telling their Stories*. Kidderminster: BILD Publications.
Duffy, S. (2003) *Keys to Citizenship: A Guide to Getting Good Support Services for People with Learning Difficulties*. Birkenhead: Paradigm.

Sanderson, H., Kennedy, J., Ritchie, P. with Goodwin, G. (1997) *People, Plans and Possibilities: Exploring Person Centred Planning.* Edinburgh: SHS.

References

Bradley, A. (2005) *Understanding Support Services for people with Learning Disabilities.* Kidderminster: BILD Publications.

Bridges, W. (2003) *Managing Transitions.* New York: Perseus Press.

Brigham, L., Atkinson, D., Jackson, M., Rolph, S. and Walmsley, J. (2000) *Crossing Boundaries: Change and Continuity in the History of Learning Disability.* Kidderminster: BILD Publications.

CSV (2006) Community Service Volunteers Royal Albert Hospital Archive: Unlocking the Past. Available at: www.unlockingthepast.org.uk

Department of Health (2001) *Valuing People: A New Strategy for Learning Disability for the 21st Century.* London: Department of Health.

Department of Health (2002) *Planning with People: Towards Person-centred Approaches.* London: Department of Health. Available at: www.doh.gov.uk/learningdisabilities

Department of Health (2006) *Our Health, Our Care. Our Say*, London: The Stationery Office.

Department of Health and Social Security (1971) *Better Services for the Mentally Handicapped.* London: HMSO.

Duffy, S. (2003) *Keys to Citizenship: A Guide to Getting Good Support Services for People with Learning Difficulties.* Birkenhead: Paradigm.

HMSO *Allegations of Ill-treatment of Patients and Other Irregularities at the Ely Hospital* (1969). Author G. Howe, Cardiff.

Mental Deficiency Act (1913). London: HMSO.

Mental Health Act (1913). London: HMSO.

National Health Service Act (1913). London: HMSO.

Report of the Committee of Enquiry into Mental Handicap Nursing and Care (Jay Report) (1979). London: HMSO (2 vols).

Kilbane, J. and Sanderson, H. (2004) 'What' and 'how' understanding professional involvement in person centred planning styles and approaches, *Learning Disability Practice*, 7(4): 16–20.

Kilbane, J. and Thompson, J. (2004) Never ceasing our exploration: understanding person centred planning, *Learning Disability Practice*, 7(3): 28–31.

Mitchell, D. (2000) Ambiguous boundaries; retrieving the history of learning disability nursing, in L. Brigham, D. Atkinson, M. Jackson, S. Rolph and J. Walmsley (eds) *Crossing Boundaries: Change and Continuity in the History of Learning Disability.* Kidderminster: BILD Publications.

Mount, B. (1987) 'Personal futures planning: finding directions for change', unpublished PhD thesis, University of Georgia.

O'Brien, J. and O'Brien, C.L. (eds) (2001) *A Little Book about Person Centered Planning*. Toronto: Inclusion Press.

O'Brien, J. and O'Brien, C.L. (2002) *Implementing Person Centered Planning: Voices of Experience*. Toronto: Inclusion Press.

O'Brien, J. and Tyne, A. (1981) *The Principle of Normalisation*. London: Values Into Action.

Pearpoint, J., O'Brien, J. and Forest, M. (1993) *PATH: A Workbook for Planning Positive, Possible Futures*, 2nd edn. Toronto: Inclusion Press.

Race, D. (1994) Historical development of service provision, in N. Malin (ed.) *Services for People with Learning Disabilities*. London: Taylor & Francis.

RHA (1983) *A Model District Service: Services for People Who Are Mentally Handicapped*. Lancashire: North West Regional Health Authority.

Robertson, J., Emerson, E., Hatton, C. et al. (2005) *The Impact of Person Centred Planning*. Lancaster: Institute for Health Research, Lancaster University.

Routledge, M., Sanderson, H. and Greig, R. (2002) Planning with people: the development of guidance on person centred planning from the English Department of Health, in J. O'Brien and C.L. O'Brien (eds) *Implementing Person Centered Planning: Voices of Experience*. Toronto: Inclusion Press.

Sanderson, H. (2000) Critical issues in the implementation of essential lifestyle planning within a complex organisation: an action research investigation within a learning disability service, unpublished PhD thesis, Manchester Metropolitan University.

Sanderson, H. (2002) Person centred teams, in J. O'Brien and C.L. O'Brien (eds) *Implementing Person Centred Planning*. Toronto: Inclusion Press.

Sanderson, H., Kennedy, J., Ritchie, P. with Goodwin, G. (1997) *People, Plans and Possibilities: Exploring Person Centred Planning*. Edinburgh: SHS.

Schön, D. (1983) The Reflective Practitioner. San Francisco, CA: Jossey-Bass.

Scottish Executive (2000) *The Same as You? A Review of Services for People with Learning Disabilities*. Edinburgh: Scottish Executive.

Smull, M. (2001) 'Revisiting choice', in J. O'Brien and C.L. O'Brien (eds) *A Little Book about Person Centered Planning*. Toronto: Inclusion Press.

Smull, M. and Harrison, S.B. (1992) *Supporting People with Severe Reputations in the Community*. Alexandria, VA: National Association of State Mental Retardation Program Directors.

Smull, M. and Sanderson, H., Person Centred Thinking in M. Smull, H. Sanderson, with C. Sweeney, L. Skelhorn, A. George, M.L. Bourne and M. Steinbeck (eds) *Essential Lifestyle Planning for Everyone*. Manchester: The Learning Community.

Tredgold, A.F. (1909) The feebleminded: a social danger, *Eugenics Review*, 1: 97–104.

Vandercook, T., York, J. and Forest, M. (1989) The McGill Action Planning System (MAPs): A strategy for building the vision, *Journal of the Association for Persons with Severe Handicaps*, 14: 205–15.

WAG (2001) The Learning Disability Advisory Group Report to the National Assembly for Wales, *Fulfilling the Promises: Proposals for a Framework for Services for People with Learning Disabilities* (LD1031) Cardiff: Welsh Assembly Government.

Wheatley, M. (2002) *Turning to One Another: Simple Conversations to Restore Hope to the Future*. San Francisco, CA: Berrett Koehler.

Wolfensberger, W. (1972) *Normalisation: The Principle of Normalisation in Human Services*. Toronto: National Institute on Mental Retardation.

2 Towards person centred practice

Jackie Kilbane, Jeanette Thompson and Helen Sanderson

Key issues

- Person centred practice
- Principles of person centred practice
- Framework of person centred practice for professionals

Introduction

In this chapter we present a framework for understanding person centred thinking and planning in relation to the role of the professional. The first section in this chapter identifies and defines key person centred terms and principles that shape person centred professional practices. These principles are located and discussed in relation to the challenges of citizenship for people with learning disabilities and the scope of professional involvement in plans and planning. In the next section, we introduce the concept of person centred practice used here and explore what is meant by this at individual, team and organisational levels. Stories and case studies emphasise the positive and possible professional contributions that make a difference to people with learning disabilities and their families in the move towards increasingly person centred professional practice.

This chapter has been written with several underpinning assumptions. These are:

- Person centred practice connects deeply with what we feel is important to and for people with learning disabilities and the professionals who come into their lives.
- As professionals, we are embedded within wider service and professional systems. This work is part of a wider configuration of beliefs, practices and behavioural norms.

- Readers will have already moved some distance towards person centred practice in their professional role/s.
- No matter how effective we are within our professional roles, using skills, talents, gifts, qualities and time, further movement towards more person centred practice is always possible.
- Making significant shifts towards person centred practice in our work reverberates not only in what we do, but in our professional identities and actions.

Building on these assumptions, we debate the critical question that forms the central theme of this book: How can we as practitioners move towards professional practices that locate the person at the centre of their life, not just at the centre of our professional interventions?

Meanings and definitions: understanding key terms

The publication of *Valuing People* (Department of Health 2001) placed an emphasis on the centrality of person centred planning in the development of services and service relationships with people with learning disabilities. Person centred planning guidance stated that, 'When we use the term "person centred" we mean activities which are based upon what is important to a person from their own perspective and which contribute to their full inclusion in society' (Department of Health 2001). Learning and developments in relation to person centred planning before and after this publication have meant that a number of different terms have emerged and are now commonly used. These are summarised now.

Person centred planning

Person centred planning discovers and acts on what is important to a person. It is a process for continual listening and learning, focusing on what is important to someone now and in the future, and acting upon this in alliance with their family and their friends. This listening is used to understand a person's capacities and choices. Person centred planning is the basis for problem solving and negotiation to mobilise the necessary resources to pursue a person's aspirations. These resources may be obtained from someone's own network, service providers or from non-specialist and non-service sources (Department of Health 2001).

Person centred thinking

Person centred thinking comprises the thoughtful application of a number of different tools that reflect person centred principles. Person centred thinking skills are the fundamental components of person centred planning. An example of a person centred thinking skill is being able to separate what is *important to* someone from what is *important for* them, and to find the balance between them (for more information, see Chapters 3 and 10). For each person centred thinking skill, there is one or more practical person centred thinking tools. An example of a person centred thinking tool is the communication chart, which is a way to record how someone communicates with us, and how we should respond (for more information on communication charts, see Chapter 7).

Person centred approaches

Person centred approaches design and deliver services and support based on what is important to a person. Hence person centred planning can promote person centred approaches. Person centred approaches are ways of commissioning, providing and organising services based on listening to what people want, to help them live in their communities as they choose. These approaches work to use resources flexibly, designed around what is important to a person from their *own* perspective, and work to remove any cultural and organisational barriers to this. People are not simply placed in pre-existing services and expected to adjust, rather, the service strives to adjust to the person. Person centred approaches look to mainstream services and community resources for assistance and do not limit themselves to what is available within specialist learning disability services (Department of Health 2001).

Person centred reviews

A person centred review uses person centred thinking skills and tools within a meeting to review progress, develop shared actions, and capture person centred information. Traditional types of review are presented in Table 2.1,

Table 2.1   Comparison of traditional and person centred review

Traditional review	Person centred review
Traditional care management reviews	'Working/not working' review
Annual day centre reviews	'Important to/for' review
Year 9 transition reviews	
Annual day centre reviews	Citizenship review
Year 10 reviews	

in the first column, alongside the person centred review styles that can be used instead. For further information on any of the person centred review approaches see www.helensandersonassociates.co.uk

Each person centred review generates person centred information that can be developed into a 'living description' of how the person wants to live and be supported on a daily basis, or can form the beginnings of a person centred plan.

Person centred practice

These are ways of working that have the person at the centre, focused on enabling the person to have what is important to them. Within this, the person is supported to move towards their dreams or aspirations in a way that keeps them healthy, safe and well. We define person centred practice as the integration, synthesis and application of key elements of 'person centredness' described above and including person centred values, approaches, planning and thinking. Person centred practice is happening when these key elements are considered and applied as a coherent whole in the context of professional work with people.

Activity 2.1

Ask your colleagues what is distinct about person centred practice from your current practice and what is similar to what you already do.

When we have asked professionals this question over the past 15 years, some professionals have said to us, 'Nothing different there. Person centred planning? We're doing that already.' We do not agree that most professionals' work with people with learning disabilities is the same as person centred planning. However, we do think that for many professionals, there will be an overlap between current practice, shaped by individual, professional and service identities and person centred practice. Box 2.1 describes the assessment process.

Box 2.1 Assessment process

Assessment is a practice undertaken by many professionals involved in the lives of people with learning disabilities and has often been compared by professionals to person centred planning. Ritchie et al. (2003) explored the differences between assessment and person centred planning, acknowledging that good assessments involve the person, are done respectfully, and can be fair and both affirming and informative to the person. The fundamental differences are:

- *Ownership* – person centred planning takes place in the person's world, at a time in their life that makes sense to them and may not involve any services at all. Person centred planning is about the person's life and what he or she wants to do. Assessment is about what the service or professional is going to do.
- *Action* – person centred planning is about doing something and making changes, beyond assessment and description.
- *Viewpoint* – within a service, the service user requiring assessment is an important and valued event in service activity. In person centred planning, the person has professional involvement as just one of many events that shape their life.
- *Scope* – person centred planning sees the person as a citizen in a community, with a whole life and rich experience, while assessment focuses upon what people may require from services.

The more that we think of person centred thinking, planning and practice as more of the same as we have always done, then it is more likely that person centred planning morphs in to exactly that, as we minimise the differences and only look for similarities. The power of person centred practice lies in these differences and our learning as professionals about what we can do and contribute to people figuring out what they want and how to get it.

Core principles of person centred practice

Person centred practice pulls together the best of what we now know about ways of working that maximise the control individuals have to live their lives as citizens and on their own terms. Principles of person centred practice are the cornerstones for understanding the application of person centred approaches, thinking and planning. The principles involve listening, sharing power, responsive action and connecting with citizenship. Each of these principles is explored in more detail below. They are written with an implicit hierarchy in mind and each principle underpins and interconnects with the others. For example, it is not possible to share professional power effectively without listening to what is important to a person first. Listening is considered first, as this underpins the other principles.

Listening

> Listening is a magnetic and strange thing, a creative force ... When we are listened to, it creates us, makes us unfold and expand.

(Ueland 1992)

Person centred thinking and planning have as a central tenet the transformative power of listening to people with learning disabilities. This principle of person centred planning has its roots in the person centred counselling and therapeutic model developed by Carl Rogers (1961). Actively listening to another person, with our full attention, can create a kind of energy between people where it becomes possible to say what really matters, what we really want in our lives, thereby taking us further towards our own awareness about who we are and what is important to us.

Activity 2.2

Think of an instance where you have talked to someone and experienced great listening. Write this instance down, noting who was there, what the environment was like, what made this listening distinct from other times when you were speaking: how did you feel, what was the impact of this feeling and experience?

Now think of an instance where you offered great listening when someone was speaking to you. If you chose an example from your personal life in the first instance, try to select an example from your working life next, and vice versa. Write down what you were doing, how you knew you were listening well, how the person speaking responded and what your feelings were.

Listening carefully often results in an unleashing of energy in the person being listened to. Person centred planning seeks to utilise that energy for movement towards a chosen direction. It is often not possible to listen deeply to another person without creating that energy or tension in a person between how things are right now in relation to where they want things to be. PATH is the tool that harnesses this collective tension in a group setting. For professionals, we sometimes contribute to this collective listening but more often than not, we spend time with a person on a one-to-one basis. With Essential Lifestyle Planning, listening is structured by asking powerful questions and listening carefully to the responses, presenting these in a clear way in a plan. It is often the facilitator's role to be the person holding the 'containers' for what is heard and then organising the information in a way that makes sense to the person and the people who want to know and understand what has been heard.

Listening in person centred planning involves earnest *attention* and *intention*. Attention to body language, words, meaning, inspirations and aspirations. Intention to understand, to know, to connect with, to make possible, to be alongside and to support a person. We listen with attention and intention because we want to create the conditions that give voice to people whose voices have traditionally been silenced or ignored. This is significant when we connect listening with citizenship. In this instance we make a deliberate effort to listen to and amplify the voices of learning disabled people. In particular, because they have been and continue to be at risk of being marginalised as citizens in our society and in the planning of quality support services that they as citizens are entitled to.

An important intention we can have when we listen is our intention to act upon what is heard. This creates a difficult task for professionals: to listen fully and appreciatively to the whole of the person, and then act upon elements of what has been heard where we have the power to positively influence. As professionals, we can listen carefully to what is being said by a person and we can come to know what is held close to a person's heart as being important. However, there is a distinction between listening as a professional with a partial role in the person's whole life and listening to a person in the context of learning about their whole life. As professionals we are interested in the person's whole life (and our interventions may indirectly impact upon a whole range of life issues), but it is our role to really connect with and listen to the part that we are trained to contribute to in our role. We listen most carefully to what we are able to act upon that will help a person make positive changes in their lives and/or their support in the context of our professional involvement.

Listening in person centred practice involves listening both to what is *important to* someone, and what is *important for* them, for them to stay healthy, safe and well on their terms. More is written about *important to/important for* in Chapters 3 and 10. In addition, a communication chart (see Chapter 7, for more information about communication charts) is a way to capture what we understand about a person from listening well to their communications.

Listening is also important in the context of how we work within teams, professional groups and as part of whole organisations. Practising great quality of attention with colleagues when they are speaking makes a great contribution to shaping team and organisational cultures so that they reflect the types of relationships that we aspire to with people using services. Creating environments that work to surface wants and preferences, hopes and direction is fundamental to person centred planning and in turn, person centred practice for professionals.

Sharing power

Person centred planning supports the self-determination of people with learning disabilities as citizens. It does this by offering ways to listen to what is important and to act upon these things, even when the person has a significant learning disability and difficulties with communicating. Person centred planning challenges power balances between people with learning disabilities and professionals. In this way, person centred planning locates the power to know what is necessary, to make decisions and to act firmly supporting people with learning disabilities. In the past, we saw that the power to know what a person needs was located with professionals, who then figure out how to meet this professionally identified need using service structures.

The doughnut is a practical person centred thinking tool that helps us to clarify our responsibilities in someone's life, and link this to sharing power. This tool can be useful to help with our thinking about what our areas of core responsibility are in relation to our work with a person, and also identify areas that are basically none of our business.

Knowing what we have the authority to act upon comes from our professional education and our experiences in role and our positions in hierarchical service structures. When we work with people who are experiencing disempowerment, it is crucial that we understand the partialness of our contribution and the benefits and limitations to this. A fundamental question to consider when sharing power is, 'How can I use what I know and do to support this person to move towards what they consider to be important and necessary in their lives?' This question relates to the importance of sharing professional power for the benefit of people with learning disabilities and understanding the seismic, systemic shift in power that is necessary for people with learning disabilities to take up full citizenship.

Sharing power is important not only in our daily work as professionals, but also in how we help others to understand positive, empowering ways of being part of professional and service structures (Box 2.2).

Box 2.2 Sharing power

Pat is a care manager who has developed experience and expertise in working with parents who have a learning disability. She is well known for this work and is sometimes asked to present papers at conferences on how to support people with learning disability who are also parents. In addition, she is asked by service managers in the area where she works to go and talk to different community teams around the city about how to support parents with learning disabilities. Many people would have seen this as a positive opportunity to further their individual career development and professional reputations. Pat did too, and at the same time she felt strongly that her knowledge and experience had come through her work with parents themselves and that this knowledge was located not with her but with the parents and families she felt she had 'learned through and with'. Pat decided that she would not present or do workshops without the contributions of the parents themselves and instead, collaborated to develop shared presentations, writing stories and insights together with the parents. Shianna was one parent who was particularly interested in this work and what could be achieved through sharing experiences of helpful professional support with others. She co-presented alongside Pat at their first big conference presentation. It went extremely well, with great feedback from the organisers and delegates. Pat and Shianna have now met with many teams to share their learning and Shianna has presented papers on her own at several of these when Pat could not attend and they made a video about Shianna's experiences. In addition, Shianna uses the materials they developed together to talk to new parents about what they can expect and ask of services.

Pat's professional profile has certainly been raised through her efforts, but her decision to share power with parents, especially Shianna, has been something that everyone has benefited from. Her chosen approach to presentations interrupted a common pattern of locating knowledge and expertise with professionals, rather than the people we are learning with and through. Pat's story does not directly link to the development of a person centred plan or utilisation of a particular thinking skill, though it does illustrate a thoughtful, broad application of person centred principles in professional work.

Activity 2.3

List two ways that you or colleagues share power with people with learning disabilities in professional work on a day-to-day basis.

There are many everyday ways that professionals share power with people they are working with. Here are some examples from professionals:

- setting time for visits and meetings around the person's preferences and routines;
- agreeing together the outcomes for the professional support, informed by any person centred plan the person has;
- using person centred thinking tools that are designed to be focused on the person.

Responsive action

Integral to person centred planning is taking action. The section on listening emphasised the importance of listening to people with the clear intention of acting upon what is heard. Taking responsive action as professionals is tricky. Most professionals work within an organisation where there are other professionals and lots of people to support. Not all these organisations are working in ways that make it easy for professionals to be more person centred in their work. Lots of organisational cultures emphasise the centrality of achieving a multiplicity of targets, attending numerous meetings, working in rigid hierarchies, reacting to crises, with power struggles between professions and diffuse accountability for action, all of which detract from our intention to work in a person centred way. We hope that the framework for professional practice we offer later in this chapter will help to make person centred practice practical and possible for many professionals.

Taking responsive action as professionals requires us to have an openness to change the way we do things so that more people have better lives through our contributions. This involves being curious about what person centred planning, thinking and practice have to offer us as we support people as well as being willing to try to do things in a way that interrupts our usual patterns of working and making interventions.

In Chapter 12, the authors discuss different approaches to taking action as professionals using Smale's (1993) work. Using these ideas, we place emphasis upon the exchange model, where there is a core assumption that the person is the expert on their own life and problems, and that professional expertise lies in helping to create a shared understanding of the person and their situation, negotiating, problem solving and co-designing solutions. We are then involved in responsive action that creates the conditions whereby people achieve fuller citizenship. Responsive action involves being clear about what we are responsible for in our professional roles with people and what is outside our sphere of influence or none of our business. The person centred thinking tool, the doughnut, can help workers become clearer about these boundaries, see Chapter 3 for more information about this.

Connected with citizenship

In this chapter we make explicit connections between person centred practice and citizenship. We see person centred planning, thinking and practice as making a significant contribution to the journey towards citizenship for individuals with learning disabilities. Person centred planning offers a process through which aspects of citizenship can be achieved; if person centred planning is the vehicle, citizenship is the destination! The thoughtful implementation of person centred planning is grounded in beliefs and actions which serve the shift in political location of people with learning disabilities from needy recipients to equal citizens in our society. We have used 'citizenship' here as a central, organising principle that underpins the shift towards person centred professional practice.

Duffy (2003), informed by the work of the Inclusion Movement, proposes six 'keys' that collectively enable us to achieve full citizenship:

1   Self-determination – the authority to control our own lives.
2   Money – to live and control our own life.

3   Direction – a plan or an idea of what we want to achieve.
4   Home – a place that is our own and a base for life.
5   Support – help to do the things that we need help to achieve.
6   Community life – an active engagement in the life of the community and the development of our own network of relationships.

Being connected with citizenship as a principle that informs work with people is significant, as it places clear emphasis upon each individual's choice and control over their life and support, the centrality of a person's own experience of and expertise in their own life and issues, and the importance of being in and part of a community. Shaping and changing our professional work so that we take responsive action that enables more people to move towards fuller citizenship positively utilises principles of person centred practice. It is possible to 'see' the keys to citizenship in other principles presented here, for example, sharing power reflects the key of self-determination and responsive action reflects the key of support.

The principles we offer here are intended to underpin and shape how people work with people with learning disabilities in person centred practice and the six keys to citizenship guide the direction and goals of professional work. Professionals work at the interface between these and other factors that guide, focus and direction of professions, such as the quality standards advocated in the Green Paper *Independence, Well-being and Choice* (Department of Health 2005).

A framework for the application of person centred principles, planning and thinking as person centred practice

As discussed in Chapter 1, the histories of learning disability services and person centred planning have long been intertwined with the development of professional practice. As we use the impetus created by *Valuing People* (Department of Health 2001) to really further the development of new patterns of service delivery and make shifts in service relationships, there is a need to think and act strategically to maximise the quality of contributions from professionals through using person centred thinking and planning. We offer person centred practice as a way to do this.

In this section, we explore what is meant by person centred practice at a practical level, building upon the model for professional involvement in planning developed in earlier work (Kilbane and Thompson 2004; Kilbane and Sanderson 2004). Figure 2.1 identifies the framework for person centred practice we use to do this. We highlight findings from the most recent substantive research into person centred planning (Robertson et al. 2005) where this is relevant and useful.

The framework illustrates four ways that professionals can become involved in person centred planning, thinking and approaches: introducing, contributing, safeguarding and integrating. Within this framework, most professionals work within service systems and thus contribute to person centred planning within organisational operations and development at three levels: as individuals, as part of a team and within organisations. In the spiral at the centre of the model lies citizenship, highlighting the centrality of citizenship when professionals make use of person centred practice to shape their involvement in a person's life.

By *individual level*, we mean a person's direct work with people with learning disabilities, their families and carers using person centred planning styles, thinking, skills and approaches. As a baseline, individuals need to be informed about different planning styles and approaches and be comfortable with directing people to further materials and resources.

By *team level*, we mean joint working between colleagues and/or within wider multidisciplinary teams, establishing practices adopted by teams or by close colleagues using person centred planning and thinking. As a baseline, teams need to have ways of making considered decisions about who takes

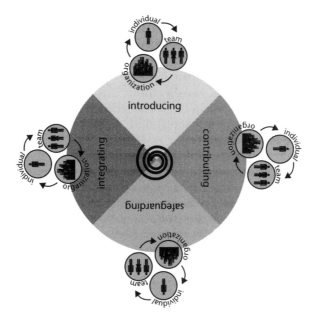

Figure 2.1 A framework for person centred practice for professionals
Source: Designed by Julie Barclay

what approach and ways of supporting and challenging each other as you learn and practice.

By *organisational level*, we mean processes and systems in place to be involved in person centred planning and practice. As a baseline, there needs to be leadership for person centred planning and practice, systems for sharing learning across the organisation and ways to decide changes to processes that are not working from the perspective of people receiving support.

Inevitably the interface between each of the ways someone can become involved in person centred planning and the different levels they contribute at are dynamic. In essence, this means that as a professional you may be introducing a person to the concepts and opportunities in planning, using person centred approaches to contribute to the planning process and be integrating learning from people's plans into the wider organisation, for example, by initiating changes in the paperwork. This would therefore also necessitate you operating at an individual, team and organisational level. The following section explores different aspects of this interface in more detail.

Introducing

At an individual level

When a person does not have a person centred plan, then a professional may introduce the idea of person centred planning with them (or their representative). If the person does want a plan, enable them to consider whether they want to gather the information themselves, whether the family want to lead the plan or with a facilitator (Box 2.3). Introducing the idea of person centred planning to an individual or their representative can happen during conversations with professionals, whether this is in a meeting or when visiting a person's home. This includes offering information to an individual about how to get started with person centred planning, supporting people to lead their own plans or how to find a facilitator.

Box 2.3 Lucas's plan

Lucas chose a student nurse to help him with his plan. He lived with three other men and wanted to move. The local self-advocacy group, People First, was running a course called 'Listen to Me' for people who wanted to use person centred planning to make changes in their lives. Lucas asked John, a student nurse he knew, to help him. John supported Lucas to think about and record how he wanted his life to be, and supported him to both arrange and speak up at his meeting, and to follow up on actions. Six months later, Lucas is now living in his own place.

Introducing person centred planning to an individual or family requires a level of knowledge about person centred planning by the professional, both in terms of understanding what it is and its styles, applications and resources. Also important within this is the local infrastructure that needs to be in place in order to support planning, such as implementation groups, courses and contacts.

Key factors to be considered therefore include:

- Professionals can help ensure that people, particularly those who are less likely to get a plan according to the research findings, have information about person centred planning and how to develop a plan if they wish to.
- Professionals can support people to lead their own plans, or work with families in this way.

At a team level

This can happen through the introduction of person centred thinking and practices to the team and thinking together about how you can make sure that everyone that the team comes in contact with knows about person centred thinking and planning.

Some tools and questions that may be of use are:

- communication charts to explore how you communicate as a team;
- 4 plus 1 questions to evaluate projects;
- growing person centred information about the team into a team plan;
- ask what you can do as a team to ensure that everyone you support knows about person centred thinking (individuals, staff teams and families).

Importantly, the more your team work in a person centred way with each other, the more effective they will be at introducing other people to person centred approaches and planning. This may be quite easy for some teams, but for others it may be a daunting task. Teams, or the people within them, are often not used to being honest with colleagues about what is important to them as well as what is important for them, or what is working and not working for them. Dealing with some of these situations can be difficult, therefore it is important to plan how you will introduce such concepts with your team if you wish to make the journey towards being a person centred team.

A 'person-centred team' is one which sees its purpose as supporting an individual to achieve the lifestyle they want as part of their local community; who are characterised by a willingness to listen and learn continually; and who highly value personal commitment and relationships with the people they support.

(Sanderson 2002b: 338)

At an organisational level

At an organisational level, this includes introducing person centred thinking and planning through the groups that professionals are involved in, and using person centred thinking within these groups, including professional networks. Each professional may be able to use their influence to introduce person centred thinking tools within the organisation more broadly. For example, if you are part of a training action group, you could introduce using person centred thinking skills there; what is working and not working from the staff, managers' and trainers' perspective about the training programme delivered in the past six months. In addition, work with the groups that you are part of to help them think about their role in enabling more people to have person centred plans.

Contributing

At an individual level

The different contributions that any professional may make to a plan include facilitating the plan (if they are trained and experienced in this), being a member of the planning process, both throughout the whole planning process or just a part of it, and contributing to actions resulting from the plan as part of implementing outcomes. In terms of practice tools, the person centred review, 'the Citizenship Review', is built on the keys to citizenship and professionals are able to usefully contribute to these. In order to contribute to a plan, a professional must be invited to do so by the person whose plan is being developed. This necessitates being clear about the focus of their contribution and being committed to completing any resulting actions.

Key implications of the role of professionals in this aspect of person centred planning include:

- Research suggests that the role of managers is a key factor in the success of plans. It is possible for professionals to collaborate with and support managers in ensuring that plans are implemented.
- Supporting people to take an active involvement in person centred planning, for example, a speech and language therapist could support people to find ways to ensure that people who do not use words to speak are enabled to be at the centre of their planning process. Again research indicates that this is a factor in positive outcomes for people from person centred planning.
- Considering training to become a facilitator. Jacob is a community

nurse with responsibility for transition. He trained as a person centred planning facilitator as he believed that these approaches were vital to helping young people make decisions about their future.

At a team level

When considering your role at a team level and what a team may offer you, it is important to think in the broadest sense about the full range of teams you are involved in. The first and most obvious is the team you are employed to work within, there are also teams built around the individuals you work with, as well as numerous other teams with a range of stakeholders. All these offer opportunities to contribute to person centred practice in a range of ways. Examples include teams exploring ways to record information in accessible styles that make it more likely that information from professionals can be included in people's person centred plans or living descriptions. Teams can also find ways to introduce person centred review processes to enhance current review practices and as a way of gathering and contributing information to person centred plans. Whatever the development area within your team, other teams you work with may find value in what you have developed.

At an organisational level

In the organisational groups that professionals contribute to, discuss and decide how more people could be enabled to have person centred plans or living descriptions. Organisations may also introduce person centred thinking tools to enhance team and organisational learning, for example, through the use of learning logs for reflective practice and supervision, particularly if the learning is generalised and the lessons learnt are implemented across the team or organisation. The acid test for any changes arising from such an approach is that they make a difference to the way we work with people who have a learning disability and to their lives.

Safeguarding

At an individual level

Professionals have a significant role in safeguarding the quality of plans and planning. Where a professional has knowledge, experience and understanding of person centred styles and approaches, they can identify where a plan is of low quality and does not reflect key features of person centred planning (Department of Health 2001). Importantly, learning from professionals about how to make plans happen can be shared with local implementation groups.

To be successful in safeguarding person centred planning so that more positive outcomes are achieved, professionals should understand key features of person centred planning, and know the elements of the different planning styles and the criteria that represent quality. In addition, it is important to be familiar with the quality process being used by the local services and the local person centred planning implementation group as well as keeping up to date with developments in person centred planning.

Key implications are:

- Professionals are in a strategic position to contribute to the safeguarding of the quality of person centred planning over time. Professionals can work with person centred planning implementation groups as a way of highlighting emerging evidence about factors that increase positive outcomes from plans, and share learning with colleagues. For example, a person centred planning co-ordinator attends the community team meeting every three months. She asks the team what is working and not working with the way that person centred planning is being implemented locally, from their perspective. She feeds this important information back to the implementation group, who use this as part of their quality process.
- Use specific research evidence to inform the focus of efforts to safeguard person centred planning, for example, learn about and share ways to support people to become active in their own plan development and make contributions to team development to increase positive outcomes from plans, and ensure that plans are available to everyone.

At a team level

The role of teams in safeguarding is crucially important, this is partly because it is difficult to set one individual up as the person who embodies the correct standards for anything, let alone person centred planning. A forum and the time to discuss quality in a general sense are therefore important. It is through the discussion and sharing of information and experiences that a shared understanding of quality in relation to plans and planning will emerge. As this emerges, each professional within the team will be better equipped to safeguard the quality of their contribution and of others in the planning process.

In addition, as the team shares information and experiences more openly through being given permission to do so, then the team as a whole becomes more person centred and more able to share those things that are important to and for them within the wider forum. Finally, as a team, it is important to ensure that plans are acted on, and the staff teams use person centred information in their daily work.

At an organisational level

Professionals who are members of organisational groups or Boards can invite the group to consider what the group's role or contribution may be to ensuring that plans are implemented and acted on as a quality safeguard. For example, a Quality Action Group did a short and focused piece of work, interviewing a random sample of people using their service, who had developed plans in the past six months, about their experiences and whether the plans had made the hoped for differences to their lives. The Quality Action Group then took action to reduce barriers to people getting the support they required that was identified through this work. In essence, therefore, organisations need to consider the infrastructures they may need or how their existing ones need to change in order to listen more closely and share power both with people who have a learning disability and with the professionals working most closely with them. Again, the acid test needs to be that something is now working differently for people who receive support from the organisation.

Integrating

At an individual level

Once a professional has experience of introducing, contributing and safeguarding person centred planning, integration of person centred planning into professional practice can happen at the individual, local and system levels also. For all professional interventions, person centred thinking and planning can be integrated into everyday professional practice by:

- spending time with the focus person and their supporters to read the plan and increase understanding of the person through the plan as part of any initial work;
- using information from plans to influence their practice, for example, arranging meetings or activities with the person in the mornings if their plan indicates this is a good time, or using learning logs;
- recording outcomes, new learning and actions resulting from professional interventions into individual person centred plans.

Using person centred thinking tools to enhance existing practices, for example, a care manager using the process called 'working and not working' in reviews, to gather information about what is working and not working from the individuals, the families and the staff perspective, when reviewing a contract.

At a team level

Fully integrating person centred thinking tools in all professional practice, systematically and habitually, rather than as a one-off. For example, using 'working and not working' in staff supervision. Teams can also review progress using the person centred thinking tool 4 plus 1 questions and using adapted learning logs instead of progress notes in records. Teams may also develop a person centred team plan that is ongoing and updated, and reviewed at team meetings. Operating in this way means that person centred practice is truly happening within the team, the culture is one of continuing to learn and develop the person centred practice of all the members of the team in an environment in which people feel safe and valued. People within the team are also comfortable and confident about sharing power with people who have a learning disability and understand the interface of their role with the six keys to citizenship.

At an organisational level
Full integration of person centred thinking skills, tools, approaches and planning in all professional practice, systematically and habitually, rather as a one-off exists across the wider organisation. Such an organisation will then be better able to recognise the value of giving people permission to reflect on how person centred they are and will integrate structures to support this in the daily ways of operating. This would also include integrating person centred principles and thinking into training and development activity, staff induction, exit interviews and the full range of opportunities associated with being employed by any particular organisation.

Conclusion

If our goal is for professionals to be truly listening, sharing power, responsive in their actions and supporting people to connect with citizenship through their interventions, all within the context of both introducing, contributing, safeguarding and integrating person centred practice at all levels within their professional and organisational structures, then we can see not only how complex the situation is but also how far we still have to travel. The first step is to believe this is truly the journey we should be taking, and we hope this chapter and the remainder of the book will provide each person with the evidence and the inspiration to take this vital step. Other chapters will also provide much more detail as to some of the practical approaches that can be taken to support this journey. At each stage of the book it will be useful to think back to the goals established within this chapter and consider how what you are reading can help achieve this ultimate goal.

Annotated bibliography

Duffy, S. (2003) *Keys to Citizenship: A Guide to Getting Good Support Services for People with Learning Difficulties.* Birkenhead: Paradigm.
The aim of this book is to help people create good individual services for people with learning difficulties, putting together the 'keys to citizenship' that are needed for people to live their own lives successfully and safely.

Kilbane, J. and Sanderson, H. (2004) 'What' and 'How': understanding professional involvement in person centred planning styles and approaches, *Learning Disability Practice*, 7(4): 16–20.
This chapter summarises a range of person centred planning styles and approaches through stories about different contributions to planning from professionals. An earlier version of the framework used in this chapter is identified and explored.

Kilbane, J. and Thompson, J. (2004) Never ceasing our exploration: understanding person centred planning, *Learning Disability Practice*, 7(3): 28–31.
This article offers a broad framework for the integration of person centred planning into professional practice and explores some of the tensions and challenges professionals encounter when using person centred planning in professional practice.

References

Department of Health (2001) *Valuing People: A New Strategy for Learning Disability for the 21st Century.* London: Department of Health.
Department of Health (2005) *Independence, Well-being and Choice: Our Vision for the Future of Social Care for Adults in England.* London: Department of Health.
Duffy, S. (2003) *Keys to Citizenship: A Guide to Getting Good Support Services for People with Learning Difficulties.* Birkenhead: Paradigm.
Kilbane, J. and Sanderson, H. (2004) 'What' and 'How': understanding professional involvement in person centred planning styles and approaches, *Learning Disability Practice*, 7(4): 16–20.
Kilbane, J. and Thompson, J. (2004) Never ceasing our exploration: understanding person centred Planning, *Learning Disability Practice*, 7(3): 28–31.
Ritchie, P., Sanderson, H., Kilbane, J. and; Routledge, M. (2003) *People, Plans and Practicalities: Achieving Change through Person Centred Planning.* Edinburgh: SHS.
Robertson, J., Emerson, E., Hatton, C. *et al.* (2005) *The Impact of Person Centred Planning.* Lancaster: Institute for Health Research, Lancaster University.
Rogers, C. (1961) *On Becoming a Person.* Boston, MA: Houghton Mifflin.
Sanderson, H. (2002a) Person centred teams, in J. O'Brien and C.L. O'Brien (eds) *Implementing Person Centered Planning.* Toronto: Inclusion Press.

Sanderson, H. (2002b) Person centred teams, in J. O'Brien and C.L. O'Brien (eds) *Implementing Person Centered Planning: Voices of Experience*. Toronto: Inclusion Press.

Smale, G., Tuson, G., Biehal, N. and Marsh, P. (1993) *Empowerment, Assessment, Care Management and the Skilled Worker*. London: HMSO.

Ueland, B. (1992) *Strength to Your Sword Arm: Selected Writings*. New York: Holy Cow! Press.

3 Person centred thinking

*Helen Sanderson, Michael Smull
and Jo Harvey*

Key issues

- What is person centred thinking?
- Why do we need person centred thinking tools?
- Practical tools for use by professionals
- Recording learning
- Organisational uses for person centred skills and tools

Introduction

Person centred planning has been evolving for a number of years and as a result of *Valuing People* (Department of Health 2001) has gained a significant profile. More recent years have seen work demonstrating the value of person centred planning, with it now accepted as evidence-based practice (Robertson et al. 2005). This has been paralleled by work to instill person centredness into the way we all approach people who have a learning disability. Fundamental to this is the range of person centred thinking skills that form the foundation of person centred planning and quality of life for people who have a learning disability. It is these person centred thinking skills that will form the basis of this chapter.

For each thinking skill, there are a number of flexible, practical person centred thinking tools. In this chapter we explore how professionals can integrate person centred ways of working within their practice. We introduce four person centred thinking skill areas and the associated person centred thinking tools. In addition, we identify ways these may be used and practical examples of how they have been used around the country. By doing so, it is intended to demonstrate how using such approaches adds to the already extensive repertoire of skills at the disposal of professionals in this area of work. In this way professionals are able to increase the impact of their work, and further increase the quality of life of the people to whom they provide a service.

Person centred thinking – what is it?

Person centred planning creates both new opportunities and new challenges for professionals. There are new opportunities to contribute to both the understanding of what quality of life means for each person and to an increased quality of life for different individuals. The particular challenges are making this goal a reality with limited time and resources. Success therefore requires 'new' skills and a critical look at existing roles. These 'new' skills are referred to as person centred thinking skills. 'New' does not mean these skills are not currently practised by many people, more that they are not yet being systematically taught to people in the context of their daily work. The skills we refer to are ones that will help professionals have better information on which to base their assessment and consultation, thus making it more likely that their recommendations will be effectively implemented.

Person centred planning has now been in use for 20 years and research has demonstrated that it does make a difference to the quality of life of people. Recent research from the UK found:

> Very little change was apparent in people's lives prior to the introduction of person centred planning. After the introduction of person centred planning, significant positive changes were found in the areas of: social networks; contact with family; contact with friends; community based activities; scheduled day activities; and levels of choice.
>
> (Robertson et al. 2005: vii)

As significant as this is, experience has also shown that it is not the mere presence of a person centred plan that makes the difference. The factors that make the difference include:

- the quality of the learning that went into the plan;
- the commitment of people around the person to implement what is learned;
- the knowledgeable support of those with power and authority.

So our goal is not to simply teach how to write person centred plans, rather our goals are to teach people how to do the following:

- Listen, learn and understand what is *important to* and *important for* each person.

- Develop person centred descriptions that synthesise and organise the learning so that it describes not only what is *important to* and *important for* each person but also describes the balance between them.
- Engage all the critical people in doing this work: the person, family members, those around the person, and managers.
- See this as an ongoing process, one of continuous learning and synthesis, rather than as an annual event.

To accomplish these goals we need to deconstruct what we were teaching in 'plan writing' and see these activities as discrete as well as interrelated skills. We then need to not only teach the skills but also reinforce their use so that they become 'habits' and part of the organisational culture.

Person centred thinking – why do we need it?

Our experience in using person centred thinking skills suggests that the use of professional time will become much more effective through the use of this skill set, thus maximising the use of a very scarce and valuable resource. As was noted, some of these skills are not new. Many professionals have stories that illustrate how they have looked behind the question asked and found a better answer. A simple example of this is Maurice's story, written by one of the authors:

> *Maurice is a soft-spoken man who is quite determined to get what is important to him. I was asked to look at his circumstances because staff were restraining him to keep him safe. Maurice lives in a climate where winter is very cold, where it is often well below zero. From time to time Maurice insisted on leaving the house that he lives in to walk to the store and would not wait for staff to drive him. Even wearing his warm winter coat he was at risk of serious frostbite. Staff had a protocol that began with them asking him to wait until they could drive him, but often that did not work. In order to stop him from leaving they often had to resort to physical restraint.*
>
> *This was the description that was initially provided and if it was all of the information that was available then it would seem that staff were justified in physically stopping Maurice in order to keep him safe. However, when the author and a small group looked at what was important to Maurice we found that a critical part of his morning routine was to have toast and jam for breakfast. To Maurice, there was no acceptable substitute for toast and jam and the group home regularly ran out of jam. When Maurice got up in the morning and there was no jam he would put on his coat and head for the door. Staff rationalised their approach by saying that it was important*

for Maurice to learn patience. Through his behaviour Maurice was saying that it was important to him to have the breakfast that he wanted.

Ignoring what was important to Maurice led to a power struggle rather than simple problem solving. Once those supporting Maurice took a step back they could see that buying two jars of jam and then replacing each when it ran out would give Maurice what was important to him. The situation went from a lose–lose situation to a win–win as Maurice had something that was important to him and staff no longer needed to try and stop him from leaving the house. From the perspective of the agency the investment in another jar of jam meant that Maurice was no longer at risk of injury from the cold or from being restrained and staff became much happier as they no longer had to enforce a rule that made no sense.

This is the 'professional as hero' story. The professional finds the simple, but profound, answer that others had not seen. But while the answer for Maurice was simple, changing the thinking that created the problem is not. The simplicity of the answer rests in a different way of thinking about people with disabilities, in looking at what is *important to* Maurice as well as looking at what is *important for* Maurice.

This is the core skill, sorting what is *important to* people from what is *important for* people, and then looking for a balance between them. Simple as this sounds, all too often it is not the reality of how services and professionals operate. Unless this skill is taught and then practised until it becomes habit, real change will not happen outside of the narrow set of situations that the professional consults on. The good news is that this is a skill that is easily taught and easily reinforced. But it must be taught, then practised and seen as valuable. For the professional some of the work of teaching and reinforcing can begin with simply asking, 'Is this *important to* the person or *important for* the person?' and then facilitating a brief discussion with others around the individual.

Informally teaching and encouraging the use of these skills becomes even more important when we realise that for every story like Maurice's, there is a counter-story. One of the authors was asked to consult with Teresa, whose challenging behaviours had resulted in multiple medications being prescribed and frequent episodes of restraint (to keep her from running into the street). When I met Teresa I saw a person that Herb Lovett would have characterised as a steadfast social critic. Until we got her supports and services 'right', she would keep telling us how wrong it was. Like many people whose behaviours challenge the system, Teresa had more than one issue. Those who supported her had to take into account the effects of her having grown up in a setting where she had been abused and typical learning about social norms and boundaries had not occurred. They also needed to consider the unusual ways in which she processed and responded to what she was told and saw and the atypical ways in which she responded to medication.

What I saw were staff who, for the most part, cared deeply about Teresa. But they had not created an environment in which Teresa felt safe (and did not see that keeping her safe and helping her feel safe were different activities). There was a lack of clarity about roles and responsibilities in a setting where Teresa was testing boundaries daily. The staff's response to many of Teresa's challenging behaviours were not working and they did not have effective ways to learn from what they were doing to discover what would work. Finally, some of the staff clearly evoked a greater number of challenging behaviours than others when working with Teresa, but nothing was being done to learn from this.

All of this was described in a report that went into detail about what the issues were and how to deal with them. The report was welcomed and praised, but little happened to change Teresa's life. Advocacy and expressions of distress had no effect. A few years later staff working for this agency had person centred thinking skill training and one of the managers became a 'coach' in person centred thinking skills (Box 3.1).

The coach used the skills taught to apply the recommendations. She used something called the doughnut sort to clarify roles. She used a matching staff tool to learn the characteristics of those who supported Teresa best. She used a set of tools that are designed to capture and analyze learning so that staff could make use of what was working and stop repeating what was not working. As a result, Teresa is happier. She is not being restrained, is on far fewer medications, and is supported by people who are a good match to her needs. Recommendations without effective tools for implementation did not work. Only when the manager had the tools that she needed to effectively act on the recommendations did real change happen.

This example demonstrates that person centred thinking tools can make the professional's role easier and more effective. As you apply, informally teach, and encourage the use of these tools, you will find that they do not replace what you have learned, instead they make it easier to apply the best professional skills that you have developed. They will help you have better partnerships with those responsible for the implementation of what you recommend. As the use of the skills becomes habit within the organisations

---

Box 3.1 Coaches

Coaches are typically front line managers whose roles include informal skill teaching. Coaching training for managers was developed as it became clear that simply doing training for direct support staff was insufficient.

that you work with, your ability to engage in best practice will increase. The following skills will help in your efforts to improve the quality of life of the people that you are working with.

Person centred thinking skills and tools

Each style of person centred planning has some foundation skills that people need to learn if they are going to create plans. In Essential Lifestyle Planning there are five basic skills and seven practical tools. These basic tools also lay the foundations for other skills that lead to building community connections and supporting dreams. In this chapter we will describe and illustrate four of these skills and their associated tools. Further information and resources about all the skills and tools can be found on www.helensandersonassociates.co.uk.

One way to think about person centred thinking skills and tools is demonstrated in Table 3.1.

Table 3.1   Person centred thinking skills and tools

Skill	Tool
Separating what is *important to* from what is *important for* and finding a balance between them	A simple grid for recording what is learned
Defining the *roles and responsibilities* of those who are paid to support	The *doughnut sort* – looking at core responsibilities, where to use judgement and creativity, what is not the responsibility of those who are paid
Getting a good match between those who are paid and those who use the services – *matching staff to the person*	A table to record what skills, supports and people characteristics make for a good match
Learning, using and recording how people communicate (especially with people who do not communicate with words)	A *communication chart* to provide a snap shot of how someone communicates
Supporting 'mindful' learning	a. Sorting *what is working and not working* from the perspective of the person and those around the person b. Using *4 plus 1 questions* to quickly and effectively record the current learning c. Using a *learning log* to record what is working and not working

In the next section of this chapter we review four of the skills and the associated tools. We will not be including the communication chart, as this is described in Chapter 7.

Sorting *important to* from *important for* and finding the balance between them

This is a fundamental person centred thinking skill. What is *important to* a person includes what people are 'saying' with their words or through their behaviour. For many people this is affected by the fact they have lived in circumstances where they were expected to say what others wanted them to say. Where people are saying what they think we want to hear, we have to rely on 'listening' to their behaviour.

What is *important for* people includes those things that we need to keep in mind for people regarding issues of health or safety, and what others see as important for the person to be a valued member of their community. This person centred thinking skill is to sort and separate what is *important to* and *important for* the person, and to find a balance between them.

The idea of the balance between what is *important to* and what is *important for* a person is rooted in the human condition where none of us has a life where we have everything that is *important to* us and none of us pay perfect attention to everything that is *important for* us. All of us strive for a balance between them. Learning what is *important to* and what is *important for* has to be done before you can help find the balance. Everyone finds what is *important to* them and what is *important for* them in conflict from time to time.

Activity 3.1

Think about what is *important to* and *important for* you, now write these down so you can refer back to them as you read the chapter. Now look at how you balance these two aspects of your life. What does this tell you about the risks and compromises you make? What does this mean in relation to the risks and balances the people you work with are able to make and to your perception of your 'duty of care'?

Finding a good balance between what is *important to* you, and what is *important for* you is often a struggle (see Figure 3.1). What we have seen over the years is that almost everyone in need of long-term services, who is in circumstances where others exercise control, has what is *important for* them addressed, while what is *important to* them is often largely ignored or seen as what is done when time permits. Those who are receiving services are often told that issues of

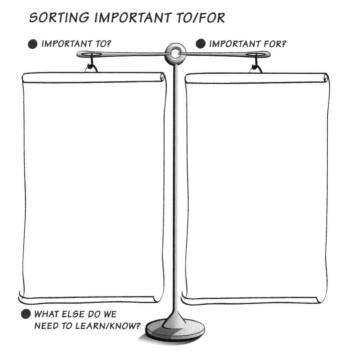

Figure 3.1   Sorting *important to* and *important for*
Source: Reprinted with kind permission from The Learning Community for Person Centred Practices and
Helen Sanderson Associates

health and safety should be *important to* them even when their behaviour
says it is not, often this is predicated on the professionals' belief that their
duty of care means that this must be so. In addition, those providing the
services are told that issues of health and safety are paramount and therefore
the significance of what is *important to* people is lost. Any intervention or
programme designed to address what is *important for* someone without taking
into account what is *important to* that person, is not adequate and often will
fail. Conversely, simply saying that we support choice and paying no attention
to what is *important for* people creates an environment where choice is used
as an excuse for doing nothing and as a result people may be hurt. Every
programme and intervention must take both into account and strive to find a
balance between them that works for the person.

Part of why those who work with people with significant disabilities must
apply this skill in their day-to-day work is not just the presence of a disability
but also the absence of control in critical areas. We should all be trying to
help people maximise the positive control they have over their lives. This
means that you are helping people find the balance between *important to* and

important for that works for them. A balance that accounts for issues of health and safety but recognises that perfect health and perfect safety are rarely achieved and all of us address what is *important for* us in the context of what is *important to* us. This is a human issue, not just a disability issue.

A doctor who specialises in sports medicine knows that advice to an injured athlete must include alternative ways to stay fit as well as what exercise not to do. The presence of a significant disability makes the effort more complex. But problem solving to find the best balance requires that people first know how to consistently separate what is *important to* from what is *important for*. It also requires that they recognise what they do not know. Those who are paid are typically operating in 'crisis mode' and may be looking for the quick fix, teams often assume that they know things that they actually do not know.

Here is a range of possible uses of *important to/important for*:

- *Assessment* When assessing people, making sure that you pay attention to what matters to the person from their perspective as well as what support they need. For example, a speech and language therapy student used the *important to* and *important for* tool at the beginning of her assessment of Jo's speech and language skills. It gave Jo an opportunity to discuss what she wanted from the assessment and what she thought the student speech and language therapist could help her with. It also helped clarify what Jo thought the assessment was about.
- *Planning and intervention* Ensure that your planning and intervention take full account of what is important to the person. For example, a care management team in Camden are encouraging care managers, support workers and people who use the service, to use the *important to* and *important for* tool within their care planning process.
- *Review* Review the impact of your work on what is *important to* the person as well as what is *important for* them. Professionals will have information to contribute to individual's reviews (for example, transition review). Increasingly these reviews are using *important to* and *important for* as ways of gathering and sharing information:

  > I very much welcomed the shift in the way this process allowed us as professionals to work, i.e. jointly and holistically rather than taking different approaches to an identified issue. I think that this shift was accelerated by the motivation generated from really hearing Yvonne's voice.
  >
  > (Speech and language therapist)

- *Reports and paperwork* Adapting paperwork that is only focused on what is *important for* the person to include what is *important to* them, for example, not just what their health issues are (*important for them*) is a really good step forward. A detailed description of what is *important to* and *for* someone is sometimes called a 'living description'. This can guide staff in what they can do to support the person. Where individuals already have a living description or person centred plan, professionals can add information to this.

- *With staff and teams* Work out what is *important to* and *for* you at work, as individuals or as a team. When you do this as a team, this can develop into a person centred team plan (Sanderson 2000).

The following example shows the *important to* and *important for* tool in operation (Box 3.2). Steven's story is an example of how the professionals in an assessment and treatment team used the *important to* and *important for* tool in their work with him and his family.

Box 3.2 Steven's story

Steven is a 59-year-old man living in a flat close to his sister and brother-in-law. Four months prior to Assessment and Treatment Services (ATSS) being contacted Steven began to demonstrate changes in his behaviour that became of concern to his family. At this time, he worked for the local council as a gardener and at work, he began to demonstrate inappropriate sexual behaviour, exposing himself in public and following some children into their home. This resulted in police involvement and Steven was arrested and released because he was assessed as being mentally unwell. He was admitted to a psychiatric inpatient setting where he was treated with 'Rispiridone' with the aim of addressing his mental illness (diagnosed at this time as a 'manic episode') and reducing his libido. During this time it became clear that the council were pursuing an incident that had taken place within work time and he was suspended from work awaiting the results of this procedure.

After a number of weeks on the ward, ATSS were contacted and became involved in the planned discharge from hospital. Work focused around assessing Steven's mood on and off the ward. He was supported to visit his sister and to slowly begin the move to home. During this process, person centred thinking tools were used with the family and Steven to enable the team (including doctors and social workers) to ensure that adequate support would be available to Steven while protecting his wish to continue living independently.

The 'important to/important for' tool was used with Steven, his sister and his niece. Steven was assessed to have a significant learning disability and associated comprehension difficulties (despite being previously unknown to all Learning Disability services). It quickly became apparent that his family had been the vital factor in enabling Steven to live and work in the community. It was identified that there was at this time a significant conflict between 'important to' and 'important for'. Steven wanted to be back at work and to live in his flat but seemed to be dazed and disorientated and less able to look after himself than he had been prior to his admission to hospital (this was established through the detailed gathering of before and after support requirements).

Steven was not able to elaborate further on important to, other than to state the importance of being allowed to return to 'Crown Green bowling' when the summer arrived but his family were able to say that it was important for him to 'have a routine' and this structure had always come from being at work. They also felt it was important to him to continue living in his flat and to be able to regain the skills and confidence he had lost. Using this information and working constantly with the family to ascertain the levels of support they were willing to offer, ATSS supported Steven to walk to town and use the bank and slowly regain his skills. This was further supported by the introduction of home care aides.

However, the biggest factor identified as being important to Steven by himself and his family was 'work'. Despite efforts to speak to his employer and to establish alternatives, this issue was not resolved. The ATSS discharged him having ensured that Steven was as well as he could be (in the absence of work) and wrote the important to and for factors into his 'staying well plan' highlighting that these issues had a direct relationship with his ability to maintain his mental well-being.

In this instance the *important to/for* tool allowed the team to support Steven and his family to begin to take some control over their situation. In addition, they were able to get their voice heard among a number of different agencies at a time when potentially the *important fors* would have dictated his future life. If this work had not been carried out with Steven and his family, then in the fallout from this episode he may well have lost his home as well as his job.

Defining staff roles and responsibilities

One of the critical skills for the implementation of person centred plans is creating clarity over the roles and responsibilities of different people. One way to do this is referred to as the 'doughnut'. The doughnut is a tool that helps staff not only see what they must do (core responsibilities) but where they can try things (judgement and creativity) and just as importantly, what is not their responsibility. Figure 3.2 illustrates this.

Activity 3.2

Think about your work role. Identify what the core responsibilities are in your role as a professional. Where can you use creativity and judgement? Share this with your colleagues and see if you have the same ideas and understanding. What does it mean if you do not have the same view, do you need to do anything about this?

THE DOUGHNUT

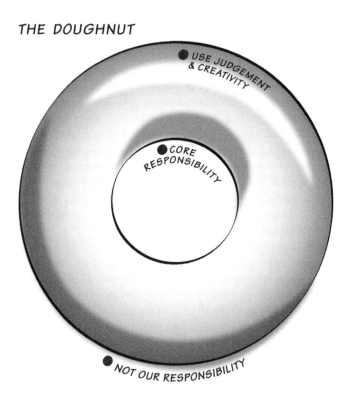

Figure 3.2 The doughnut

Source: Reprinted with kind permission from The learning Community for Person Centred Practices and Helen Sanderson Associates.

You and your colleagues may have different ideas about what your core responsibilities are and where you can use creativity and judgement. In some situations this will not be problematic, however, if the differences are substantial, you may find it useful to carry out the doughnut exercise as a team of professionals to ensure the best use of the available resources.

Using the doughnut enables staff to know where creativity is and is not expected, and within those boundaries to be creative without fear. This is important as there will never be enough funding to provide people with all the things that are important to them. Where there is not enough money, we need more creativity. We need the creativity of the person and everyone around them to maximise outcomes. An additional advantage of clarity around roles is that of accountability. Where boundaries are clear, you are reinforcing accountability. Great services hold people accountable for their performance inside those boundaries. Using the doughnut helps provide a foundation for that accountability.

Whenever the people who work within an organisation are unclear about how to sort their responsibilities, the doughnut should be introduced and used until everyone is clear about the expectations for performance within their jobs. There are different ways that the doughnut could be useful in working with staff and teams. One possible way is to help staff to think about what their core responsibilities are in implementing a plan/programme, and where they can use creativity and judgement. This could also be used within your professional team, clarifying what your core responsibilities are and where you can use creativity and judgement. For example, one care management team manager used the doughnut with a steering group looking at a service restructure: '*This helped us focus on our core responsibilities and how they could be retained throughout the change process.*' Other people have used it as part of the supervisory process that supports professional activity.

Activity 3.3
Can you think of any other ways of using the doughnut to support professional practice or organisational development?

You will probably have identified a range of possible uses, one that we are aware of was when a team of multidisciplinary health professionals chose to explore a real-life situation they were faced with in their work, using the doughnut sort.

The psychiatrist in the team shared the person's story with the rest of the group. They were supporting a young man who had severe diabetes, which needed to be managed by both insulin and an appropriate diet. The team had worked hard to support the young man with his diabetes, helping him to understand the importance of his diet in the management of his condition. However, the young man loved junk food and would consume large amounts of it on a daily basis. This led to his diabetes being very unstable and him being very ill at times. He had already lost some of this toes on his left foot and the team were concerned about his future health if he continued to eat junk food and ignore the dietary advice they gave him. They were very clear that he understood the consequences of what he was doing when he was eating the junk food and how it affected his health.

The team used the doughnut sort to clarify their thinking around the situation, after much discussion they agreed the following:

- Core responsibilities – they felt it was their core responsibility to ensure that he had all the information he needed about diabetes and how his condition needed to be managed through his diet. They also felt it was their core responsibility to provide him with information about the likely consequences if he did not manage his diet. All of this information needed to be presented to him in a way that he could understand and it was their core responsibility to make sure this happened.

- Judgement and creativity – they felt that they could use judgement and creativity about how they presented this information to him, i.e. the formats used to ensure he completely understood the consequences of his actions. They discussed how different types of advertising about giving up smoking, for example, work for different people and the team discussed some ideas about how they could present the information to him in creative ways.
- Not our paid responsibility – the team felt it was not their paid responsibility to stop him eating the junk food and ignoring their advice.

Using the doughnut sort enabled each professional and the team to be very clear about where their responsibilities lay with regard to this issue. It also helped them to identify some new things to try in the way they presented the information to the young man. In addition, the doughnut sort had helped them to explore their 'duty of care' in a safe and structured way.

Matching staff and those using services

One of the most powerful determinants of quality of life for people who use services is the match between them and the people who provide support (see Figure 3.3). Figure 3.3 is a simple way to record what is needed to give you the 'best match' between those who use services and those who provide them. This can also be represented in grid form. Whatever approach is used, the most important part of this is the part where personality characteristics are recorded. When organisations look at the skills needed to support someone, they typically limit themselves to the skills needed to address issues of health and safety and the general skills needed for the position. In completing this form, those who fill it out should also address the skills needed for someone to have what is *important to* them as well as what is *important for* them. While having the right skills is a minimum expectation, the match regarding characteristics is critical. When we are talking about skills in this context, we are including any skills needed to help people have a balance between what is important to them and what is important for them. Where there is a good match between those who are paid and those who receive services, there is less turnover.

Having the skills that address the balance between *important to* and *important for* and the personality characteristics needed, helps create a match between the person using the services and the person providing the services. This is a win-win situation for everyone. From the perspective of the person

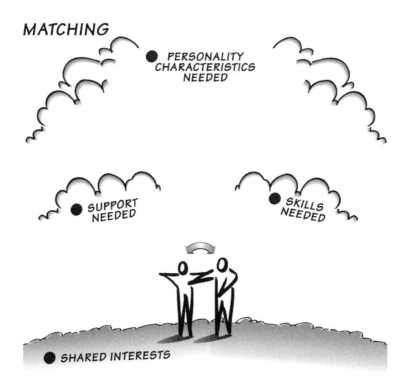

Figure 3.3 Matching staff and those users services
Source: Reprinted with kind permission from The Learning Community for Person Centred Practices and Helen Sanderson Associates.

receiving the services, having someone with the right skills and the right personality characteristics greatly enhances the quality of life, regardless of the presence or absence of a person centred plan. From the perspective of the person providing the support, they are being paid, however inadequately, to have fun in a role where they feel competent.

From the perspective of the organisation, having this kind of match could reduce turnover as people who provide the services are getting to do what they do best. When skills and personality characteristics are matched, the frequency of challenging behaviours should decline along with incidents of abuse and neglect.

Activity 3.4
If you were looking for someone to live with you, as a lodger in your house, what would you be looking for? Use the matching staff format to identify the skills they would need, the personality characteristics and the shared hobbies that would make as near a perfect fit as possible!

If you have ever shared a house with someone who was a 'bad match', you can see how important this tool could be! A 'bad match' situation can lead to a range of outcomes, feeling insecure, inadequate, a propensity to violence and general physical ill health, to name but a few.

While a number of organisations already do much of this matching work on an informal basis, many feel they need support in using this tool more formally. Others will agree that it is a good idea but will tell you it will not work for them. Given the clear and powerful benefits that these efforts provide, it is not surprising that the resistance comes from an equally powerful place. Where people are served in groups and a small number of paid staff work with a larger number of people, these efforts are often seen as interesting but not applicable. They do not see how they can make improvements without changing their core structures. Where professionals work within organisations that have such perceptions, you need to help them look at how they move forward incrementally. See if the match can be improved for more people even if it cannot be improved for all. Where there is a particularly bad match, see if the problem is how people are being grouped together and seek to find ways to give people more control over who they live with. Recognise that it is part of a different way of thinking. If you are successful in helping people think differently, then the organisation will be willing to work on changing how it supports people.

Here is a range of possible uses of 'matching staff':

- Supporting a staff team to think about which member of staff would be best suited to supporting a service user.
- Applying the same principles to recruiting a new team member to a therapy service or multidisciplinary team.
- A care manager supporting a family in recruiting someone to work with a family member, using direct payments.
- Working with a staff team around someone who has the label of challenging behaviour to work out the best match of team members to the individual to help to reduce challenges. For example, an Assessment and Treatment team in Derbyshire have developed team profiles for each member of the team, detailing their gifts,

talents and interests. When a person is referred to the service, they or those that know them well are shown the profiles and meet the team members and then they decide who will be best to work with that person.

How Simon and his care manager used the staff matching grid

As part of a planning session to help Simon identify the support he needed to purchase with his individual budget, a care manager used the matching staff grid (Table 3.2) to help him think about the qualities he required in those supporting him.

The following information from the grid was then included in Simon's support plan and used as a basis for his support:

- I need my support worker to be good with my money and benefits while still making sure I am involved.

Table 3.2 Simon's matching staff grid

Supports wanted and needed	Skills needed	Personality characteristics needed	Shared common interests
Help to develop independent living skills around the home	Cooking – understanding of healthy eating Cleaning Washing		
Support to go out in the community and develop new interests, i.e. joining clubs, football matches	A good community connector	Enthusiastic Good listener	Computer games X Box Board games Likes football and preferably supports Arsenal!
Prompting with personal hygiene		Sensitivity Empathy Support but not over-caring	
Support with managing money	Budgeting skills	Supportive but not controlling	
Support with medication	Basic medication training	Sensible	

- I need support to stay healthy and safe. My family and others around me worry that sometimes I am at risk; I need support to stay safe.
- I don't want to feel like I have a 'carer', I don't want other people to see me being 'looked after'.
- I need support and prompting with personal care and some everyday living skills.
- I need support to learn how to prepare healthy meals and have a balanced diet.
- I want to be involved in choosing my own support workers.

Skills and qualities Simon stated his supporter should have:

- My supporter should be a good listener.
- Some of my support will be around my home helping me to set up routines and develop my living skills.
- I will also need to get support to get out and about in the community and make friends. I need someone to help make friends and meet people my own age. My supporter must be willing to join in with me in clubs or groups until I have made some friends.
- My supporter will need to prompt me and guide me with my personal hygiene, helping me learn how to look after myself and set up a routine.
- I would need support to help me learn to manage my money so one day I can be in total control of it.
- I need support to learn about any medication I might need to take in the future, as I once took an overdose and I am worried this will happen again.

Being 'mindful' and recording learning

Structured, 'mindful' learning is critical to ensuring person centred practice and that person centred plans are implemented. Having plans that change as understanding deepens, and as the person changes is crucial. As is having the information which tells us the point at which services and supports need to change. In this chapter we will discuss three different tools that operate within this skill domain. The three tools are:

- working/not working
- 4 plus 1 questions
- the learning log.

Working/not working

This is an analytic tool that supports you in looking at a snapshot in time from multiple perspectives. It is a way to analyse a situation so that you capture what is working or making sense within that situation as well as what is not working. In appearance it is quite simple. One of its functions is to see where there is consensus from different perspectives and where there is disagreement. The tool can also help to build action plans by identifying what is necessary to sustain what is working, and what it would take to change those aspects of a person's life that are not working (Figure 3.4).

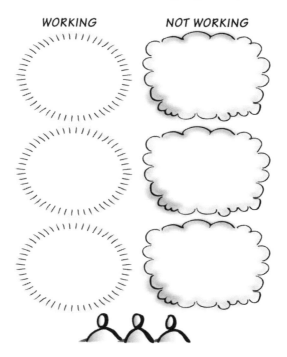

Figure 3.4   Working/not working

Source: Reprinted with kind permission from The Learning Community for Person Centred Practices and Helen Sanderson Associates.

The following demonstrates some of the possible ways in which 'working/ not working' can be used to help existing systems become more effective:

- In reviewing progress with a service user and their family about an intervention or support package. For example, an occupational therapist used working/not working with someone who uses a wheelchair, so that they could evaluate together how the new wheelchair was working out, from both their perspectives.

- In team meetings to reflect on a project, for example, the care management team in Camden have used the working/not working tool to review their duty system.
- In meetings around an individual to look at what is working and not working from the person's, family's and other team members' perspectives.
- In care management reviews, see Box 3.3.
- In transition and other reviews (see Chapter 9).
- In staff supervision.
- In supporting staff and families where there are difficulties in getting a shared understanding on an issue, see Box 3.4.

Box 3.3 Care management review

Care managers in Camden developed a new review format. This looks specifically at current services and whether they are still meeting the service user's community and health needs. The tool being tried is the 'what's working, what's not working' model. The service user's views are expressed first in each section, with others' views taken into account. The reviewer uses a 'learning log' to record how well they thought the review worked and suggestions for future reviews. The review format is to be sent out prior to the review. This process is becoming much more of a 'self-review'. Initial feedback has been positive. Some users have found the process unfamiliar and have found it difficult to answer some of the questions. Care managers state: '*We believe that this is because many have never been asked for their own views on their lives and services, and we hope that this will in itself be a more empowering experience.*'

Box 3.4 Support for Helen

Helen has been planning with her supporters for six months, she lives in a small community mental health hospital having moved from a large hospital in 2003. Helen has decided that she wants to move on and live more independently. However, Helen did move before but the placement broke down as Helen found it difficult to take her medication. Helen and others are anxious about this, so it was discussed at a planning meeting. Using the working/not working format, the following was agreed:

- Blister packs do not make sense to Helen – they look the same whichever way up they are – success would be unlikely.
- Helen loves colours and these may help make sense of her medication for Helen. She loves pink and purple.

- The team agreed to try to find or make a medication box based on colours for Helen to use.

Although the team recognised that Helen would still be dependent on someone putting her tablets into the correct compartments, it is hoped to work on creative solutions to this in the future.

The 4 plus 1 questions

This is a simple but powerful tool for professionals. (Figure 3.5). The four questions are:

1   What have you tried?
2   What have you learned?

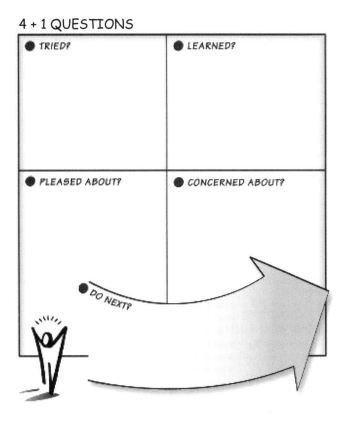

4 + 1 QUESTIONS

| ● TRIED? | ● LEARNED? |
| ● PLEASED ABOUT? | ● CONCERNED ABOUT? |

● DO NEXT?

Figure 3.5   4 plus 1 questions

Source: Reprinted with kind permission from The Learning Community for Person Centred Practices and Helen Sanderson Associates.

3   What are you pleased about?

4   What are you concerned about?

The questions are useful when meeting in order to gather the team's collective learning in a way that leads to answering a fifth question:

5   Based on what we know, how should we move forward?

Here is a range of possible uses of 4 plus 1 questions:

- In reviewing progress with a service user and their family about an intervention.
- In team meetings to reflect on a project, for example, a physio-therapist used the 4 plus 1 questions as part of the review of a dys-phagia group. For each individual who attended the group they explored the four questions. This led them to agree what they would do next. The physiotherapist said that it helped them to focus on how dysphagia affects the person rather than the actual swallowing problem.
- In meetings around an individual to look at what is working and not working from the person's, family's and other team members' perspectives.
- In care management planning and reviews, for example, care managers are using the 4 plus 1 questions as part of the care planning process. They state: *'Support staff and families are being encouraged to use these tools to plan not just for services that the local authority can provide, but also to develop their own pathways to improving their quality of life.'*
- In transition and other reviews.
- In staff supervision.
- In supporting staff and families where there are difficulties in getting a shared understanding on an issue.

The learning log

The learning log can be used to replace some traditional notes or records. The idea is simple. Where learning should be taking place in the course of an activity, provide a way for those engaged in the activity to record what they have learned – focusing on what worked and did not work. Learning logs were developed so that staff could record learning but have since been adapted so that those who are using the services can record their learning as well. Figure 3.6 shows one of the most common formats for a learning log. This version was developed in Oregon and works well to record the learning of staff. The version in Figure 3.7 was developed in the UK and works equally well in recording the learning of the person using the services.

Charlie's Learning Log

Date	What did the person do? (What, where, when, how long, etc.)	Who was there? (Names of staff, friends, others, etc.)	What did you learn about what worked well? What did the person like about the activity? What needs to stay the same?	What did you learn about what didn't work well? What did the person not like about the activity? What needs to be different?
3/1	Hillsboro Aquatic Center for hot tubbing (2 hours)	Charlie, Aaron, John, Trina and two strangers	He liked the long warm soak part. The hot tub temperature is set at 105 degrees, which is not too hot for Charlie. Charlie especially liked floating on his back with Aaron's support. We saw lots of smiles and a very relaxed Charlie.	Charlie did not like getting rain on his face when we were getting in the van. We need to take an umbrella when we go out on rainy days. The lift was not available when we arrived at the center. Call ahead next time. (503-648-9884)
3/4	Fishing at Hide a-way resort (2.5 hours)	Charlie and Aaron	He liked catching the trout and got so excited he didn't want to leave. Charlie liked the hot cocoa + cookies we shared.	We need to figure out a way for Charlie to hold his pole more on his own.
3/5	Neighborhood walk (30 min)	Charlie, Trina, Aaron	Charlie likes to greet the dog at the corner of 5th and Jersey. We stopped about 10 minutes each time we walk.	Today we tried to go a different way. Charlie was not happy until we turned around and went down 5th 1st. Take a dog biscuit next time!
3/5	Reading with his new glasses (1 hour)	Charlie and Mrs. Endicott	Mrs. Endicott and Charlie read a fishing magazine "Northwest Fishing". He loved having Mrs. E. to himself for a little while! They had lunch together also. The glasses really help Charlie see the pictures.	He was not interested in the car magazine she brought. Not sure if it was because he was hungry or because he wasn't interested in cars.
3/6	Shopping in downtown with a walk (1.5 hours)	Charlie, Don, and Judy	Charlie got very excited and yelled out a few times when we were looking at video games, at Electronic Salon. A Woman in the book store took special interest in Charlie and helped us find books on fishing (at Dottons).	Construction at the mall downtown (Pioneer Square) made our time not as fun. There were lots of detours + narrow paths and the smell of some fumes made Charlie's eyes water and caused some discomfort.

Figure 3.6 A learning log
Source: Reproduced with kind permission from The Learning Community for Person Centred Practices and Helen Sanderson Associates.

things I have been doing

Date	What I did	Who was there?	What was good?	What was not good?
	Think about: • When it was • Where it was • How long it was for	Think about: • Did you like them being there? • Who else would you have liked to be there?	Think about: • I liked ..... • I felt ......, • I want more ..... • I learned	Think about: • I did not like ...... • I felt ......, • I want less ..., • I learned

Figure 3.7 Learning log for the person to complete
Source: Reproduced with kind permission from Helen Sanderson Associates.

Typical notes found in the records of people who use services are intended to document what was supposed to happen and what did happen. In those instances where learning is recorded, it is often buried in a long narrative. Those who are doing the day-to-day work with the person are learning and often what they are learning is critical information about the person. But because that learning is either not recorded or not recorded in an accessible format, it gets lost. The learning leaves when the staff member leaves. The people in Oregon developed the learning log when they heard what Amy's nurse had learned. Amy hated medical appointments. The nurse who worked with Amy recorded what happened at her medical appointment but not what she did to help Amy cope with waiting. Rather than have Amy wait in the doctor's office, she took her through a 'drive through' car wash. Amy, who did not communicate with words, was happier and more excited in the car wash than anyone had ever seen before. The creative and skilful way that this nurse supported Amy was not part of her nursing notes until the learning log format was developed.

Acting on this kind of learning can have a substantial impact on the quality of life for people with severe disabilities using services. However, it can happen only if the learning is valued, recorded and acted on. Sadly, it is rare that we ask people who use services to record their learning, even though many people are capable and interested in doing so. For those people, the second format (Figure 3.7) gives them a way to do so.

The following are some additional uses of the learning log:

- Asking a staff team to record notes about a specific intervention/ programme instead of progress notes, for example, in the 'Hours Work Project' all teams use learning logs for clients. For 20 people in total, learning is summarised once a month and entered onto the recording system. Case notes sheets have been replaced by learning logs.
- Therapy assistants using the learning log to record their sessions with clients.

Using person centred thinking to inform organisational change

In this chapter we introduced four person centred thinking skills and their associated tools, and provided possible ways that they could be used by professionals. In addition to using them to enable change at an individual level, they can also contribute to our learning about how the organisation needs to change. For example, in one area, the person centred planning co-ordinator attends the therapist's team meeting every two months. She asks them to think about the people that they have worked with over the past month, and, from their perspective, give an idea of what is working and not working in those individuals' lives. The specific issues are captured, for about ten individuals, without using their names, and this information is fed to the person centred planning implementation group as one part of intelligence gathering about the service.

At the implementation group meeting, they do a cluster analysis of what is working and not working in the lives of around 40 people who use services. Each cluster is then named, for example, what is working well may include people who are taking part in activities in their community, or people having their own tenancies, and what is not working may include people being bored at the day centre, inconsistent staff support or people living with others that they do not like. This gives an indication of what is working and not working in the service, that can point to where the implementation group needs to learn more, where they can act to strengthen or increase what is working well, where they can change what is not working, and what is outside their sphere of influence that needs to be shared with the Partnership Board. In this way, professionals simply using 'what is working and not working' to think about some of the individuals that they are involved with, contributes to the learning about what needs to change in an organisation.

Conclusion

Person centred thinking skills and tools have the potential to make the professional's role easier and more effective. As we have said earlier, they do not replace what you have learned; they simply make it easier to apply best professional skills and practices. As these tools are more commonly used within services they create a new shared language for support staff, managers and professionals. This can strengthen and enable better partnerships. In services that have embraced this way of working, you hear conversations about whether something is important to or important for the person, about whether something is working or not working, and whether something is a core responsibility or an area where the staff can use their creativity and judgement. These tools can be used within multi-agency teams, to explore what is working and not working for the team, or to clarify core responsibilities and creativity and judgement. And, finally, as we have shown, they also provide additional ways to influence organisational change and development, particularly using working/not working for individuals, and exploring what this tells us needs to change in services, and using 4 plus 1 questions to reflect on projects and initiatives.

Acknowledgements

We would like to thank the following people for contributing to this chapter by sharing their stories and examples:

- Neil Woodhead – Person Centred Planning Co-ordinator Derby Assessment Treatment and Support Service, Derbyshire Mental Health Services;
- Stuart McMullen, Debbie Thurlow and Camden Care Managers;
- Janet Bartle – Person Centred Planning Co-ordinator, Berkshire Healthcare NHS Trust;
- Helen Millett;
- Hours Work Employment Project;
- Stockport Good Great Team;
- Amy Duck, speech and language therapist, Camden.

Annotated bibliography

Helen Sanderson Associates (2006) *Person Centred Thinking Minibook*. Manchester: HSA Press.
A minibook compiled from *Essential Lifestyle Planning for Everyone* by Helen Sanderson and Michael Smull, identifying each person centred thinking skill. This book is available as a free download from www.helensandersonassociates.co.uk

Sanderson, H. and Smull, M. (2001) *Essential Lifestyle Planning for Everyone*. Manchester: HSA Press.
Since first developing essential lifestyle planning in the late 1980s/early 1990s, the authors have continued to learn how to better develop plans that helped people who use disability services get the lives that they wanted. This edition of the handbook moves from a focus on plans with people with disabilities, to plans for everyone who wants one. What we teach and how we teach change as we learn more about what needs to be present in order to develop good plans that make a difference.

References

Department of Health (2001) *Valuing People: A New Strategy for Learning Disability for the 21st Century*. London: Department of Health.
Robertson, J., Emerson, E., Hatton, C. et al. (2005) *The Impact of Person Centred Planning*. Lancaster: Institute for Health Research, Lancaster University.

Sanderson, H. (2000) Critical issues in the implementation of Essential Lifestyle Planning within a complex organisation: an action research investigation within a learning disability service. unpublished PhD thesis, Manchester Metropolitan University.

Useful resources

The Learning Community for Essential Lifestyle Planning
www.learningcommunity.us

Helen Sanderson Associates
www.helensandersonassociates.co.uk

Person Centred Thinking Templates
www.helensandersonassociates.co.uk

Valuing People Support Team
www.valuingpeople.gov.uk

4 Person centred partnerships

Simon Duffy and Sam Smith

Key issues

- The fundamental partnership for the professional should be the one they forge with the person they serve, and other partnerships should support this primary relationship
- The purpose of partnership is to enable people to be full and active citizens and person centred planning provides a range of helpful tools for the person to achieve citizenship
- The current system for delivering support is inappropriate and assumes that professionals will control the support that disabled people receive; instead people need to be able themselves to control the support they receive
- C-Change for Inclusion is a support organisation that shows how a real partnership can be built between the person and professionals using person centred planning
- C-Change for Inclusion and the people it serves also benefit from the wider partnerships that have been constructed to support learning and inclusion

Introduction

When we use terms like 'partnership' or 'integration' in the public sector, there is a tendency to focus on the variety of ways in which different public bodies are able to come together and co-operate (Hudson 2005). But if we are not careful, these organisational partnerships can distract us from examining the real partnership that needs to be at the core of any professional's work, their own relationship with the person they serve (Duffy 2004). It is in the creation of a partnership here, between the person and the professional, where the real challenge and the real possibility of good practice lie.

Person centred planning provides an exciting set of tools for building partnerships where power is returned to where it belongs, into the hands of disabled people. Even those people who are most easily marginalised and excluded, the people who are sometimes said to have 'challenging behaviour' or 'complex needs' can all benefit from an approach which takes our individuality and need for self-determination seriously.

In this chapter we will explore the nature of this fundamental partnership between the person and the professional and explore the case of C-Change for Inclusion, an organisation that demonstrates both how it is possible to ensure everyone can be in control of their own support, and the value of other organisational partnerships to achieve this aim.

Citizenship

Partnership is not an end in itself and to explore the concept of partnership we need to begin by considering its central purpose. Disabled people themselves have described that purpose powerfully in a number of ways, for example, the National Centre for Independent Living describes its purpose as *'to enable disabled people to be equal citizens with choice, control, rights and full economic, social and cultural lives'* (www.ncil.org.uk). Central England People First's aims include *'to make sure that people with learning difficulties know about their rights, can get their rights and have the same rights as everybody else'* (www.peoplefirst.org.uk).

For government too, the general direction of policy at both the local and national level has increasingly begun to focus on citizenship. For example, in England this policy was set out in the *Valuing People* White Paper (Department of Health 2001). A clear indication is given in this document regarding the lives of people with learning disabilities and their families and carers, and how they should improve, based on recognition of their rights as citizens, social inclusion in local communities, choice in their daily lives and real opportunities to be independent (Department of Health 2001: 10).

In Scotland, a similar policy direction was detailed in *The Same As You*.

> *In future, both children and adults with learning disabilities should, wherever possible, be supported to lead a full life with their families or in their own homes . . . it should allow them to live a full life and be included in society while providing privacy and allowing them to develop.*
>
> (Scottish Executive 2000: 39)

At the same time, emerging from the field of professional practice, concepts like citizenship were being used to build on the work of O'Brien and others and to demonstrate how practical innovations like person centred planning, supported living and direct payments all linked back to a simple but powerful concept of everyday citizenship.

Activity 4.1

Why is citizenship important to people who you work with that have a learning disability?

Duffy has used the idea of citizenship as a core concept in helping disabled people, their families and professionals think about how best to design individual support services and ensure that people are protected from exploitation and enabled to live full lives:

> *Citizenship matters because we are different. The very fact that we are different makes us vulnerable to prejudice, exclusion and segregation, as the history of disability shows. But a commitment to citizenship gives us the chance to fight the human tendency to exploit the disadvantages of others. This will never be simply a matter of changing a law or of reorganising services. We will need to be constantly alert to the possibility that others are being cut out of community.*

(Duffy 2003: 165)

As this book demonstrates, person centred planning has a particularly valuable role to play in supporting people to be citizens and it does so in a number of ways. We can see this if we divide Duffy's analysis of citizenship into six keys and examine how person centred planning helps orientate people towards citizenship. The six keys are:

1 Self-determination
2 Direction
3 Money
4 Home
5 Support
6 Community life.

Self-determination

Self-determination is our ability to make our own decisions about our own lives. Person centred planning is a way of returning the power to make decisions back to people who have been deprived of that power and including even those whose communication skills seem very poor or those where it is not clear how much they understand. Person centred planning overcomes these problems by offering multiple ways of listening to what the person wants and understanding who the person is.

Although very different in style, the search in PATH for the dream of the person and those who love the person shares the same goal as the behavioural analysis of communication methods we find in essential lifestyle planning. Each is a focused effort to attend, not just to the words we use, but to our bodies, our moods, even our half-articulated desires.

This also explains why much of the training in person centred planning focuses on helping people create an environment where the individual can be heard. In fact, particular planning techniques are rarely as important as ensuring that the person feels central to the discussion and can control their involvement. Good person centred planning is creative self-determination in practice.

Activity 4.2

How can you support a person you work with to have control over the decisions that are made and hence their own life?

Direction

The second key to citizenship is having our own personal direction, a sense of who we are and where we are going in life. Although this may seem rather esoteric, personal direction is actually critical to our sense of self-worth and personal identity. To have no direction is to be lost and to be without a way of anchoring your relationship to other human beings.

Again, person centred planning techniques are all methods for finding direction, whether that is through positive open questions about expressing gifts or following dreams, or through critical evaluative questions about what is making sense or is not making sense in our life. It is only with this central analytical tool that the person centred planning process can create the necessary dynamism for future action.

Moreover, the need for direction also explains why person centred planning cannot be value neutral. Effective planning requires those who are planning to assume that each individual has their own unique positive value and that listening to the individual positively will help the person find their own path. Such an approach will not make sense for someone who does not believe in the innate worth of all human beings and the value of diversity.

Money

The third key to citizenship, money, seems far removed from person centred planning, almost at odds with it. In fact, the PATH planning process begins by encouraging people to dream with no reference to money, to avoid being artificially tied down by preconceived notions of what is possible.[1] In reality, good person centred planning involves not being shy about thinking about the place of money in our lives nor the necessity to think about money when making changes to our lives. Good planning must always come back to an active engagement with constraints, particularly as those constraints will also provide opportunities.

In fact, it is even possible to argue that the recent policy developments in England that have promoted personalised budgets have arisen precisely because national progress in person centred planning was being constrained by the block purchasing of standardised social care services by local authorities and the NHS.[2] Too often those who have been planning have been told that any radical change is impossible, not because what they wanted was more expensive, but because it required funding to be 'released' from pre-purchased services.

Home

The fourth key to citizenship is having your own home, a place where you can control who you are with, a place where you belong and a place of retreat and personal privacy.

Activity 4.3

How might not having a tenancy or a home you can have control in, affect your ability to achieve self-determination and a good life?

People who do not have a home are always vulnerable, always subject to the power of others. Often the importance of a home is discovered as we listen to people plan. It is frequently one of the things that people want to change in their life, particularly because the high rates of institutionalisation in the UK mean that disabled people are usually 'housed' but rarely in their own homes.

Good person centred planning can become a very practical tool for helping people find their own home. For instance, Nan developed a personalised menu of housing options, with her friends, before deciding to set up home with her friend Christine (Duffy 2003). In 1999, Link Housing in Edinburgh helped people successfully close a residential home by supporting every-body to do their own person centred plan and identify a better home for themselves.

Support

The fifth key to citizenship is to receive support from others. This does not mean support in the narrow sense of disability support services. We all need support from others, or we will become detached from other human beings. A community of equal citizens is not a group of people who need nothing from each other, rather, it is a community of mutually dependent people with needs and duties to each other. For people without a disability, getting support from others is a normal and everyday part of life, usually governed by family relationships, social relationships and commitments or by commercial exchange. If, however, you require support because of a significant disability, you are liable to find yourselves heavily dependent upon others and less able than others to direct that support.

Person centred planning is one critical element in helping to achieve self-directed support, support that enhances rather than frustrates citizenship, because person centred planning helps people identify what support is really for, and how best to deliver it. This can be seen particularly in essential lifestyle planning, which draws special attention to the question: 'How do we success-fully support the individual?' This simple question is critically important for people who cannot use words, money or power to let you know what kind of support they want. It is only by attending, with great care to the very particular support needs of the individual that the professional can properly fulfil their role.

Community life

The sixth and final key to citizenship is our active contribution to the life of our community. In fact, it is arguable that most of the early work in person centred planning, particularly Mount's work on personal futures planning, was primarily driven by the desire to demonstrate how disabled people could be helped to make their own contribution to the life of the community (Mount 1987).

Activity 4.4

How does your job as a professional help people contribute to their community? How might you do more of this in your role?

Mount's work helped people reflect differently upon the opportunities that lie locked in our communities and within ourselves and which are sometimes only unlocked when we pay positive attention to what we can do and what is available from others. The idea of 'mapping' these possibilities – writing them up on large charts, exploring connections, refusing to be limited by the obvious service – has played an enormous part in helping people problem-solve more effectively.

So, in summary, citizenship is a valuable way of determining the purpose of our lives and that of our professional practice when supporting others. Good person centred planning can support citizenship in the following ways:

- demonstrating self-determination in practice;
- helping people find direction in their lives;
- helping people maximise and make the best use of their money;
- helping people identify the right home for themselves;
- identifying both the purpose and quality of good support;
- creating a vision of a full and productive life.

The obvious corollary of all this is that these objectives cannot be achieved by the professional alone. Person centred planning is the individual planning their own life, with the support that is right for them. So the professional will need to radically reconsider their role in the life of the person who is planning. They may still have a role, but that role must be based on partnership with the person.

Another way of thinking about this challenge is to see that we cannot 'do citizenship *to* someone'. For citizenship to be meaningful, it has to come *from* the person. Even if we could provide all the conditions necessary for citizenship: autonomy, a plan, money, a house, support and a community, it is only when these conditions are 'activated' by the individual that citizenship will be achieved.

It is this fact that demands a very different response from professionals, for when citizenship is the goal, then the professional cannot act alone. The professional has to become a partner with the individual, working to help them articulate and achieve those aspirations which build citizenship. Unfortunately the current organisation of services is designed neither to support the development of positive partnerships, nor to achieve citizenship.

The power balance

The most fundamental challenge for human services, if they mean to help rather than hinder people's achievement of citizenship, is to change the fundamental power relationship that presently exists between professionals and the disabled people they serve.

Human services have been built around the professional gift model of service delivery, which assumes that needy individuals will be given what they require by the professionals who understand those needs (see Figure 4.1) (Duffy 1996). Operating within this paradigm it seems natural for human service professionals to be in control. However, there is a significant risk that operating in this way will lead to the individual being treated as the object of professional help (Oliver 1996).

However, this does not have to be the model we use to deliver human services. Increasingly, systems of support are shifting away from professionally

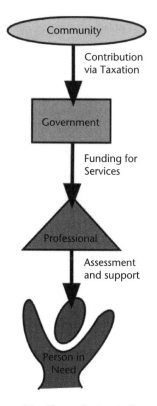

Figure 4.1 The professional gift model

dominated systems towards self-directed support, where disabled people themselves control how they live and the support they need (O'Brien 2001; Glasby and Littlechild 2002; Leadbeater 2004; Poll et al. 2006). This new and emerging paradigm might be called the citizenship model of service delivery (see Figure 4.2) (Duffy 1996). In this new paradigm the individual is at the centre of defining their own life and their own place in the community. Critically, resources are no longer given to professionals so that they can provide services on their terms; instead the individual's needs entitle them to the resources necessary for them to live their own life. The services they receive are negotiated between them and any professionals they choose to use.

Clearly, achieving such a significant paradigm shift is not straightforward, and there are further complexities to explore when there are duties of care towards the individual or where the individual needs help with making their own decisions. However, we can already identify some of the major steps necessary to make the shift. The case study that follows (Box 4.1) describes how one organisation, C-Change for Inclusion, has begun to define its own role in terms of a partnership with the disabled person to help them achieve citizenship. We will also go on to see that this first and critical form of partnership has a significant impact on how the organisation goes on to build other forms of partnership.

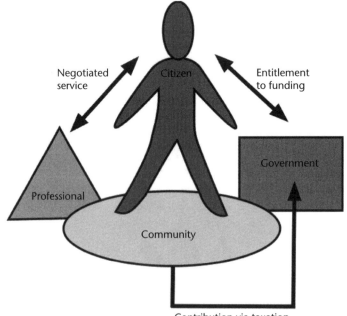

Figure 4.2 The citizenship model

Box 4.1 C-Change for Inclusion

The story of C-Change cannot be told without reference to Inclusion Glasgow, an organisation started by Simon Duffy in 1996. Inclusion Glasgow had been challenging the traditional models of support offered in the Glasgow area (Scottish Executive 2000). The organisation supported people to live where they wanted, with whom they wanted and with control over their day-to-day support. It also had a commitment to remain small and community-based and by 2000 it had reached its self-imposed maximum size by supporting 50 people. At the same time the local authorities were aiming to finally close Lennox Castle Hospital, at one time the largest institution in Scotland, but now containing approximately 200 people, most of whom were considered to have complex physical support needs or were perceived to be 'challenging'. Inclusion Glasgow wanted to continue to help people move on from this environment but instead of expanding its own size, it offered to host the development of another service provider, C-Change for Inclusion.

C-Change began life on 1 May 2001 with the twin aims of supporting people who would otherwise have remained excluded from the community and providing support in an affordable and person centred way. Sam Smith, the Director of C-Change, described her reason for starting the organisation as follows:

> *While working as a Commissioner in the Glasgow Learning Disability Partnership I became aware of a commonly held view that supported living was possible for most adults with learning difficulties but expensive, and therefore unaffordable, for anyone who was deemed to be 'complex' or 'challenging'. One of the aims when establishing C-Change was to dispel this myth.*

The organisation was designed and structured to provide 'robust' person centred services for adults and young people with learning difficulties or mental health problems who would otherwise remain in secure or excluded settings. The aim was to confront the prevalent assumption that people who challenge services should remain in congregate living arrangements where their behaviour could be 'managed'. Instead C-Change was founded to provide support that puts the disabled person at the centre of the service and ensures that they are in as much control of the day-to-day decision-making as possible. The hypothesis was that if the organisation listened more, was more adaptable and recognised mistakes sooner and rectified them faster, then it would be able to show that people who 'challenge' can be supported to live within their communities with an affordable level of funding. This assumption was based on the fact that many of the challenges that people presented were caused by the services that they received and that sometimes too much support could be as harmful as too little.

Inclusion Glasgow was already providing a template for how to successfully provide highly individualised services, yet many of the professionals who were responsible for services in Glasgow were challenged by its ethos, style and policies. Working in this person centred way involves taking risks and challenging long-held assumptions about the potential of people with very negative reputations. It was therefore imperative that a way was found to build active partnerships with families, advocates and professionals and to avoid being isolated when taking necessary risks or developing innovative supports, so C-Change worked especially hard to build a commitment to partnership into its structures and processes.

C-Change frequently starts working with people when they are living in segregated or secure settings. These environments are not conducive to person centred planning. People living in deprived or restrictive living environments frequently have limited expectations about the possibilities that will be available to them when they move. Equally, the professionals involved in supporting people in institutional settings may have limited experience of community living and may find it difficult to see the potential and scope for change in the person they work with. In these circumstances it is very easy for people to become stuck: constrained either by their own fears or the fears of those around them. In the remainder of this chapter and Boxes 4.2–4.5 we will describe how C-Change for Inclusion did not allow that to happen, how it worked to make sure that everybody was able to benefit from citizenship and control over their own life. To describe how this was done, we will tell a few stories that represent different aspects of the challenge of achieving citizenship and creating meaningful partnerships.

Box 4.2 Imran's story

Imran's story exemplifies the hurdles that different perspectives on personal potential and risk can raise. Imran was to move out of a secure hospital ward into his own home, but the professionals from the hospital found it hard to believe that Imran could be safely supported in his own home. They suggested that Imran needed five staff with him at all times, based on the fact that it took five staff to restrain him in the hospital when he became upset. Their thinking was based upon their experience of supporting Imran in a hospital ward with 24 other residents. Imran's mum was very keen for him to move out of hospital and to be nearer to her. She had no experience of supported living and was extremely worried about Imran's move, thus she supported the suggestion that he should have five staff with him at all times. However, C-Change found it difficult to accept that it would be helpful for Imran to have five people working with him at all times.

The hospital psychologist, psychiatrist and nursing staff worked with their community-based equivalents, with Imran's mum and with the C-Change team to come up with a compromise that respected these different perspectives. Imran moved into his own home with three staff supporting him at all times for the first month (with one person always staying in a separate room), this was then reduced to two staff and finally to a service based upon one-to-one support with 12 hours of additional flexible support per week to be used as required. This process of service design and planning enabled differing perspectives to be considered and respected and ensured that Imran's needs determined how his support evolved.

In practice, helping Imran meant building trust between different people even when there was disagreement. It is not enough to be right, it is much more important that Imran gets the chance to lead a better life. This took compromise and a willingness to listen and learn on all sides. This is the critical first step to person centred work: to be prepared not always to be right.

Box 4.3 Gregor's story

Gregor was only 19 when C-Change started working with him. He had lived at home with his family for most of his life, but the situation at home was difficult and sometimes Gregor became frustrated and angry and would hurt his family. He moved out of the family home into his own flat, receiving support from a community outreach team. This arrangement lasted less than 12 weeks before the service broke down. The police were involved and Gregor was placed in an assessment unit.

Gregor appeared to be a very angry young man and he was also labelled as being 'on the autistic spectrum'. Gregor felt that he was not being listened to. He did not like attending meetings as he felt that these were opportunities for people to talk about him and all the things that had gone wrong in his life. He also did not like it when meetings were held without him as he did not trust what people were saying about him. He often said that he felt that things were done to him, not with him. Initial meetings with Gregor would last less than five minutes before a table would be turned upside down and he would leave the room. The challenge for C-Change was to work out what Gregor wanted to do with his life so that his support team could assist him to achieve it.

C-Change worked with Gregor for approximately six months before embarking on any structured or formal person centred planning. It was felt that Gregor needed time to recognise that his team would listen to him and act upon what he said. He needed to build trust and feel safe before anyone expected any more of him. After approximately six months, Gregor and his support team needed more direction and it was felt that only Gregor could provide this. The challenge was to engage Gregor in a person centred planning process despite the fact that he did not believe that he would be listened to and did not want to participate in anything resembling a meeting.

To find a way of listening to Gregor, C-Change focused on Gregor's gifts. Gregor has an amazing memory, particularly for music trivia. He particularly likes music quiz shows on the television, so Gregor's planning day was modelled on a particular quiz show. Gregor and his dad were the quiz masters and they made up the questions ahead of time. There were two teams, who had to answer questions posed by the quiz masters. When a team got a question right, they won the opportunity to make a suggestion for Gregor's life in the year ahead and place it on one of the planning areas on the wall: holidays, employment, relationships, community, home and garden, etc. The team would win an extra point if Gregor accepted their suggestion and it was kept in his plan. Failure to get a question right could result in the team having to sing a karaoke number of Gregor's choice.

Gregor's first planning day lasted three hours, followed by a meal enjoyed by his family and friends. Gregor did not leave the room once in anger. The person centred planning process gave Gregor and his team a plan to work towards for the year ahead. Gregor's plan detailed where he would like to go on holiday and with whom, what kind of job he would be interested in looking for and what kind of things he wanted to spend his spare time doing. Most importantly, Gregor felt listened to. The process was unconventional but it was right for Gregor. This planning day was his first step towards self-determination.

Prior to the planning day Gregor and all those involved in his wider network of support, his care manager, community nurse, psychologist, his psychiatrist and his family were all extremely anxious about the sustainability of his support service. The breakdown of his previous individual support service after such a short period of time had led to fears that Gregor could not be supported to live in the community. Gregor did not invite any of the other professionals involved in his life to his first planning day, and this caused them a degree of concern. There was an assumption by some that, given the risks, they were entitled to attend the planning day; however, the professionals were able to manage their anxieties, to step back and to allow Gregor to set the direction. This was achieved because Gregor's wider network of support had worked hard at developing a good partnership based upon trust and mutual respect.

Following the initial planning day, the role of the care manager changed. It was no longer necessary to direct Gregor's support service, Gregor did this himself, instead their role was to hold C-Change to account for supporting Gregor to achieve the plans that he determined, a role that Gregor understood and appreciated. This change in role depended upon mutual trust and respect.

Today Gregor no longer holds his planning days with a theme. He does not feel that he needs to. He books the venue and organises the agenda, he invites whom he likes and sends out the invitations. Gregor now invites some of the professionals involved in his network of support to his planning days, he does this because he wants them to be there. Gregor controls every aspect of his planning day; Gregor is in control.

Person centred planning can be a very powerful way of supporting a person to voice their ambitions and to achieve self-determination. However, it is important to recognise that person centred planning is a journey, not a destination; if the individual who is the focus of the plan is not engaged, then the process is meaningless. The individual has to be supported to direct the process, no matter how slowly and carefully.

Box 4.4 Catherine's story

One of the key mechanisms that C-Change uses to ensure that services continue to meet the changing needs of the individuals they support is the Individual Service Fund (Fitzpatrick 2006). When C-Change begins working with someone, the first step is to gather information from the individual, their family and the professionals involved. This is used to inform the budget that determines the size of the Individual Service Fund, which is the money that an individual uses to fund their support.[3] This fund can be used flexibly so that the support can be changed as the individual's needs, wishes and desires change and as the person adapts to life outside the institution. Person centred planning is used to ensure that the person controls how their service develops.

C-Change became involved in Catherine's life when the organisation supporting her felt that they could no longer work with her. Catherine had moved house many times in the previous five years and felt unable to return to the home she had at the time. Catherine found it frightening to look to the future; her main worry was where she was going to sleep at night. C-Change supported Catherine to find temporary accommodation in hotels and flats while trying to work out a longer-term plan. The uncertainty of these arrangements left Catherine feeling vulnerable and insecure and she often acted in ways that led to her losing her home. Catherine was angry with her supporters, she felt she had been let down and that she was not being listened to. Catherine would call her care manager at the Area Learning Disability office, the housing office, the C-Change office, her local hospital or her GP and express her anger. The police would sometimes be asked to intervene. Catherine was banned from most of the offices of the professionals involved in her support and some of these people would not see her on their own. Catherine was extremely vulnerable and unhappy. The challenge for C-Change was to support Catherine to feel that she could take control of her life despite the chaos she was experiencing and her lack of trust in the services that supported her.

Catherine did not have any family, but she had a network of people including her C-Change team, her community nurse, the practice team Leader, her psychiatrist, her GP and the manager of the emergency nursing team who wanted her to gain control over her life. This network developed a shared vision of the life that Catherine could live if she could be supported to see beyond the immediate difficulties she was experiencing. This network was made up of people who were willing to work together to hold the vision when things got difficult. They worked together to ensure that no one was blamed when difficult situations arose. Catherine was fortunate to have a group of individuals who were willing to commit the time to come together to participate in person centred planning in a way that made sense for her. They made the effort to listen to Catherine when she told them what she wanted and, most importantly, they did not pretend that they had all the answers. This partnership of committed individuals worked hard to gain Catherine's trust and to reassure her that they were there to listen and learn. Person centred planning played a key role in achieving this.

Catherine first experienced person centred planning at her planning mornings. These occasions were used to celebrate Catherine and her achievements, her survival skills and her generosity. Catherine's support team prepared her for these meetings, but Catherine still thought that the meetings were to discuss the problems she was causing. Catherine was disconcerted when people talked about her gifts and strengths. It had been a long time since Catherine had heard people say good things about her; she would sometimes get angry in these meetings and leave the room, but she always came back.

Things did not change quickly for Catherine; with her life in chaos she was extremely vulnerable. Those involved in her support were concerned about her welfare but knew that things would only really change if she was in control of the direction her life took. Some attempts were made by professionals who were not directly involved in her support network to take control of her life and her support by defining her expressions of distrust, upset and anger as a medical problem. The process of person centred planning gave those involved in her support network a clear picture of what Catherine saw as her future and this provided legitimacy to withstand these attempts at professional interference.

Catherine truly began to take control over the direction of her life when she got her own home in an area that she knew and where she felt safe. The Housing Association was involved in planning with Catherine and supported her when she indicated that she did not feel ready to take on the tenancy of her new home. C-Change and the Housing Association drew up a management agreement between themselves instead. There was an understanding that Catherine would assume the tenancy when and if she was ready and that she would let everyone know. Catherine is now celebrating her second year in her house and although it has not been easy for Catherine or those involved in her support, everyone has learnt a great deal along the way.

For a long time Catherine wanted to have support workers with her at all times, as she did not want to spend any time on her own, although those who knew her well felt that she was able to do so. Sometimes she would dismiss her team members on the spot and it could be difficult to recruit people to work in her team, and as a result, Catherine's Individual Service Fund was overspent. Catherine found this difficult, as she is an extremely honourable woman and does not like to be in debt to anyone. She would often say 'I like to pay my debts'.

C-Change started supporting Catherine to understand the implications of the choices she was making by working through the detail of her Individual Service Fund and how she was spending it. As soon as Catherine understood that her fund was overspent, she resolved to do something about it. She decided that she could, after all, spend time on her own. When she has a disagreement with a member of her team, the implications of 'giving them the sack' are discussed with her. If she is determined that she does not want them to work with her any longer, she knows that she has to pay them during their notice period and the implications that this will have for her fund.

Catherine is far happier having this level of control over the way her support is delivered and her service is a clear example of the opportunities that can arise through financial constraints, as Catherine said to her service manager, 'I am happy with the time on my own, you were holding me back.' Catherine now has the time and space in her life to give as well as receive support and all those who know her benefit from this. She is an inspiration to others. Catherine's story demonstrates the power and effectiveness of both listening to the person and the way in which that listening and learning can be used to build a community around the individual.

Glasgow Learning Disability Partnership: Robust Services Project

C-Change now supports 39 people to live in their own homes, alone or with someone they choose to live with. With the exception of three individuals who require some additional support, everyone receives one-to-one support, no-one supported by the organisation has two-to-one support at all times. Many people spend time on their own or in the company of friends and family. C-Change has worked hard to support people to overcome the reputations that had been assigned to them.

However, these successes were not created by C-Change alone. A significant part was played by the Glasgow Learning Disability Partnership. This was set up by the Greater Glasgow Health Board and Glasgow City Council to facilitate joint strategic planning and commissioning of learning disability services in the Greater Glasgow area. The Partnership recognised that the majority of people it funded who were labelled as having challenging behaviour and who lived in segregated services could live in the community if they received the right support. It also recognised that organisations working with these individuals would need additional support in order that risks could be managed creatively and that the services did not become prohibitively expensive.

Activity 4.6

What support structure and partnerships do you think would be useful to an organisation like C-Change if one were to start operating in your local area?

The Glasgow Learning Disability Partnership worked with three provider organisations – C-Change for Inclusion, Community Integrated Care and Turning Point – to set up the Robust Services Project in 2001. The aim was to foster true partnership working between organisations supporting individuals who had the most significant reputations for challenging the services that supported them. It was envisaged that there would be opportunities for joint learning and that this could be disseminated as best practice within the Glasgow Learning Disability Partnership. The project established a Robust Services Management Group attended by the senior managers of the provider organisations, commissioning managers, the head of profession for psychology and the manager of the Additional Support Team (a team of health professionals that provided professional input when services were at risk of breaking down). It also set up a Practice Development Group attended by service managers from the organisations involved including the managers of the assessment and treatment units run by the partnership. These groups provided an opportunity for professionals working within different cultures to share their knowledge and experience.

On a practical level the Robust Services project developed shared training, agreed risk management strategies, agreed approaches to inter-agency communication around accident and incident reporting and the components of good working policies or support plans. A less tangible but equally important benefit was the opportunity for individuals and organisations to be honest about the difficulties encountered when supporting people who are complex and challenging. Without the support of the Robust Services Project, C-Change would have found it far more difficult to continue supporting some people to live in their own homes. Harry's story is an example of how such partnership work supported a significant change of direction in the life of one individual.

Box 4.5 Harry's story

Harry had been in and out of institutional care since his early teens. Over the years a number of services, including individual services, had been commissioned for Harry and had subsequently broken down as a result of the challenges that Harry presented to those who supported him. When Harry was living in a hospital, he would challenge staff and say that he wanted to live in his own house. When he was in his house, he did things that resulted in him being re-admitted to hospital. Harry put himself and others at risk of serious harm and the police would frequently be involved. It was clear that this was a destructive cycle; the difficulty was how to break this pattern and support Harry to see that there were other directions that his life could take.

C-Change supported Harry to move into a house that had been purchased by a local Housing Association with his particular needs in mind. A working policy was drawn up that detailed the support strategies that would be used in the event that Harry challenged the service in any of the ways he had in the past. This document was agreed and signed off prior to Harry's discharge. When Harry started harming himself, the team followed the working policy; when he set fire to the house, another predictable risk, they did the same. When Harry started destroying his property, the team knew what to do, they also followed the working policy guidance when he threatened to harm them. When Harry challenged the team in unpredictable ways, by going on hunger strike and undertaking a dirty protest, the multidisciplinary group that had been meeting regularly to review Harry's service asked the Robust Services Management Group for guidance. A second opinion was also sought from the Mental Welfare Commission, they agreed that the support plan and risk management strategies being implemented were adequate and appropriate.

The multidisciplinary group working to support Harry knew that the easiest option would be for him to return to hospital. They also knew that this would merely be repeating the pattern of his life so far. They knew that as soon as Harry was admitted to hospital, he would ask to leave. It was difficult for everyone to hold to the vision, particularly when Harry's behaviour resulted in the police being involved. As a result of the commitment to multidisciplinary working and the support of the Robust Services Project, Harry did not return to hospital although he did spend two short periods in prison. Harry has been living in his own home for the past two years with no incidents of any significance. More importantly Harry no longer talks about returning to hospital. The pattern had been broken.

The Robust Services Project offered an opportunity for organisations to work together in an atmosphere of mutual respect and shared understanding and without this, C-Change would have struggled to continue to support Harry as the risks were too high to manage in isolation. Had there not been a clear framework, connecting all the key professional groups and the other service providers, then it would have been easy for C-Change to be criticised by other professionals, the police or other community groups. Instead this structure enable difficult decisions to be scrutinised and agreed and for the organisation to be defended in its work. Without the support of the Glasgow Learning Disability Partnership, and in particular those involved in the Robust Services Project, C-Change would not have been able to succeed in supporting Harry.

Altrum

C-Change has also benefited from its membership of Altrum, a very different kind of partnership organisation. Altrum is a federation of separate, diverse and creative organisations that share a common overriding purpose. Altrum's name comes from the Gaelic word meaning 'to foster' and its role is to develop its own members and nurture new organisations. It was established in 1999 on the premise that like-minded organisations could work together for mutual advantage and for the benefit of disabled people. Altrum has a number of member organisations, including C-Change, Circles Network, Diversity Matters, Elcap, Freespace, Inclusion Glasgow, Neighbourhood Networks, Paradigm, The Thistle Foundation and Partners for Inclusion and one individual member who is the parent of a young man with a disability. Members of Altrum have a set of shared values and work to reflect these values in the everyday work of member organisations. All members of Altrum agree to offer each other mutual support in a high trust environment which enables the development of best practice.

There are several practical advantages to this form of inter-organisational partnership working, one of which is that member organisations avoid pointless competition. They also share the benefits of remaining small while gaining the advantages of being part of a larger organisation when negotiating for contracts such as personnel support or training. Altrum is also able to represent the views of smaller, more creative organisations at a national policy level due to the collective size of the organisation. The work of Altrum has not only supported the ongoing work of its existing members but has been instrumental in the development of two new organisations: Neighbourhood Networks and LEAF. Altrum has also led the way in establishing a new qualification for social care workers in Scotland that is more relevant to supported living, the Higher Education Certificate in Person Centred Approaches for Social Care Workers. Membership of Altrum has enabled C-Change to develop its work over the past five years by providing a forum where like-minded people can test out ideas, challenge each other and collaborate to better meet the needs of individuals they provide support to and to enhance the primary partnership with the person.

Conclusion

The stories from C-Change help us to see that it is possible for professionals to form a positive partnership with disabled people. This will only happen, however, if that partnership is founded on a recognition of the innate dignity of all disabled people and their right to full citizenship. In addition, these stories vividly display some basic truths that we should all take cognizance of:

- Imran shows us that positive change is possible even when people are scared and in disagreement, as long as people are prepared to identify a first step towards greater trust.
- Gregor tells us that the individual must determine their own destiny and that we can help them to gain control if we concentrate upon their gifts and capacities.
- Catherine needed people to have a vision of a positive future where she could take responsibility, and once she had grasped it, exercising that responsibility was not a burden, it became a right she enjoyed using.
- Finally, Harry teaches us the enormous importance of having faith in the person, despite all setbacks; not blind faith, but faith that is the result of careful observation, reasoning and reflection.

A partnership that is based on a commitment to human dignity, to the rights of disabled people and a belief in the ability of all disabled people to make a contribution to community life, is a partnership worth developing. It is also a partnership that will help construct the kind of community that welcomes disabled people as full citizens.

Notes

1   But this initial refusal to be constrained when dreaming should not be confused with any general unwillingness to get to grips with reality. Once the dreaming stage of planning is over, the objective setting and all the other steps should be constrained by an ambitious sense of what is positive and possible.

2   For example, the research carried out on person centred planning by the University of Lancaster and others stated that '*Commissioners were struggling to identify individual sources of funding within budgets dominated by block contracts*' (Robertson et al. 2005). It was to overcome these kinds of problems that the Valuing People Support Team set up the in Control Partnership in 2003 (Poll et al. 2006).

3   In Imran's case there was some disagreement about the level of support that he required; this is particularly common when the person has a reputation for challenging services and there are concerns about the risks involved. On these

occasions C-Change may draw up a non-recurring budget, which provided additional funds that can be used to provide additional staffing through the process of transition, without committing to this level of staffing or expenditure on an ongoing basis. This can be a useful mechanism to allay the anxieties of those involved while ensuring that the needs of the individual are kept at the centre of the service design.

References

Department of Health (2001) *Valuing People: A New Strategy for Learning Disability for the 21st Century*. London: HMSO.

Duffy, S. (1996) *Unlocking the Imagination*. London: Choice Press.

Duffy, S. (2003) *Keys to Citizenship: A Guide to Getting Good Support Services for People with Learning Difficulties*. Birkenhead: Paradigm.

Duffy, S. (2004) in Control. *Journal of Integrated Care*, 12(6): 7–13.

Fitzpatrick, J. (2006) Dreaming for real: the development of Partners for Inclusion, *Journal of Integrated Care*, 14(1): 27–34.

Glasby, J. and Littlechild, R. (2002) *Social Work and Direct Payments*. Bristol: Policy Press.

Hudson, B. (2005) Partnership working and the Children's Services Agenda: is it feasible? *Journal of Integrated Care*, 13(2): 7–12.

Leadbeater, C. (2004) *Personalisation through Participation: A New Script for Public Services*. London: Demos.

Mount, B. (1987) *Person-Centred Planning*. New York: Capacity Works.

O'Brien, J. (2001) *Paying Customers Are Not Enough: The Dynamics of Individualised Funding*. Lithonia, GA: Responsive Systems Associates.

Oliver, M. (1996) *Understanding Disability: From Theory to Practice*. Basingstoke: Macmillan.

Poll, C., Duffy, S., Hatton, C., Sanderson, H. and Routledge, M. (2006) *A Report on in Control's First Phase 2003–2005*. London: in Control Publications.

Robertson, J., Emerson, E., Hatton, C. et al. (2005) *The Impact of Person Centred Planning*. Lancaster University: Health Research.

Scottish Executive (2000) *The Same as You?* A Review of Services for People with Learning Difficulties. Edinburgh: Scottish Executive.

Useful resources

NCIL
www.ncil.org.uk

People First
www.peoplefirst.org.uk

in Control
www.in-control.org.uk

5 Person centred approaches to educating the learning disability workforce

Jeanette Thompson and Lynne Westwood

Key issues

- Citizenship
- What people want from their life
- Values, knowledge and skills required of the future workforce
- What people who have a learning disability want from people who support them
- Future options for training and developing the workforce
- Person centred practice and professional courses
- Individual-led practice
- Continuing professional development and person centred practice

Introduction

This chapter is set against a backdrop of rising expectations from people who have a learning disability and significant policy changes that reflect increased choice, a louder voice and shared risk with people who need support. If the aspirations of people and those outlined in the policy documents (Department of Health 2005, 2006) are to become a reality, then the workforce development agenda has a crucial role to play. Failure to consider the implications of such changes for the workforce will only lead to compromise in the vision. The challenge therefore within this is in identifying what this agenda means for professional and vocational qualifications and what changes would be required within these areas, to ensure those who wish to access such opportunites are able to do so.

In order to answer this, it is important to focus upon the future as any changes made to established structures, such as professional and vocational qualifications, need to be rooted in longer-term strategic viability and in the needs of the population that the workforce serve. In order to do this we felt the most appropriate starting point would be to consider what the lives of people who have a learning disability might be like in the future, and what support, if any, they would want from paid staff. Having identified this, we then set about exploring the skills this group of people might need as well as the necessary knowledge and skills required to fulfil their role. Essentially we considered the workforce development needs of the people who would be employed to support people who have a learning disability in the future. This was seen as particularly important with the changing agenda resulting from the growing popularity of the self-directed support model.

In addition, it was deemed necessary to identify where we currently are in the education and development of the learning disability workforce and the wider group of people that they may have contact with. In order to identify what is important for people who have a learning disability now and in the future, we first of all considered what people in general feel is important to them.

What is important to you?

Working with a group of 60 participants (Thompson and Westwood 2007) indicated that the following areas are important to overall health and well-being:

- family
- being healthy
- work
- money
- home
- stress
- leisure
- having a history
- having something you want to achieve
- celebrating 'differentness'
- independence.

These areas were confirmed as important to people who have a learning disability when the same activity was repeated with them.

- *Family* – was seen as important in that people typically wanted to be close to their family, however they chose to define that, and to have access to them as well as a sense of belonging. Some people also felt it was important to have a sense of being useful to their family as well as their family being useful to them. This is essentially the reciprocal nature of relationships. Reciprocity is also relevant to friendships. Valued and reciprocal relationships are seen as particularly important in maintaining both an individual's physical and mental health (Grant 2005).

- *Being healthy* – is extremely important to most people. As a concept it often shifts, depending on the individual's health and their perceptions of this at the time. For many people being healthy is *not* a goal in its own right, it exists to support us to do other things. For some people being healthy is about being able to cope with the physical and mental demands of life and having a sense of purpose and direction. Souza (2006) discusses the fact that a meaningful life is important to being healthy, as without a reason to get up in the morning, health has little value.

- *Work* – is a well acknowledged determinant of people's health and well-being, alongside their status in society (Acheson 1998; Department of Health 2001, 2006). Work can also be important because it provides opportunities for us to better ourselves and to learn new things, constantly challenging our minds and bodies. In addition, it gives us the potential to earn money that helps us to live the life we choose.

- *Money* – can support us in spending time with our family and friends. It provides the means to move about in our community. For some people this area may be contained and may be the immediate geographical area in which they live. For others, their extended families and friendships may mean extensive travelling. Sustaining such relationships would not be possible without money.

- *Home* – is one of the basics in life that many of us take for granted. It is where people feel most safe and secure. Where people feel in control and do what they want, when they want, within the constraints created by living with other people. One important aspect of having a home of your own is the pressures and responsibilities that go with this. For some people those pressures are a reaffirmation of who they are and why they are important to their friends and family.

- *Stress* – is not an obvious area to identify as important in life, however, it is also well documented that appropriate levels of stress can be healthy (Selye 1956). Conversely, it is equally documented that high levels of stress can be damaging to health and well-being, therefore maintaining a balance in life is important for all of us.

- *Leisure* – an important stress buster. Each person has their own preferences about how they spend their leisure time. Some people enjoy being in their garden, others enjoy travel while others prefer the theatre or cinema. Whatever a person's preference about how they spend their leisure time, it is an important way to recharge batteries and maintain a sense of well-being.

- *Having a history* – not often something we think about, but our history denotes much of who we are and gives us a sense of place. While you may not recall telling someone your history, you may have told many different people part of your life story, clearly indicating how important it is (Rolph et al. 2005; Hewitt 2006).
- *Having something you want to achieve* – goals are crucial in life. They act as a motivator; give us a reason for being and for going to work. The things each individual wants to achieve are different. Most of us have more than one goal for a range of areas in our lives. Having a range of things to work towards is healthy. It is often what gives us our motivation to keep going with all the more mundane things in life.
- *Celebrating our 'differentness'* – again, not something we think about on a regular basis, yet we all acknowledge that we are different. At the same time, how much time and energy do we invest in trying to conform and achieve a degree of sameness? For some people, however, celebrating their 'differentness' is an important aspect of their lives, as are humour and the feeling of being alive. Often being able to spend time with someone who shares some aspect of your 'differentness' can be very helpful in relation to a person's sense of well-being.
- *Independence* – one of the commonly expressed aspects of independence is the ability to do what you want when you want while being conscious of the effects your choices have on other people.

In essence, each of the key areas listed above has a vital contribution in relation to our roles, how we are valued and our existence. These areas are essential prerequisites for feeling included, equal and not discriminated against.

Activity 5.1

Having read this information, which areas are important to you? Now think about someone you know who has a learning disability and what they would say is important to them. How does their experience compare to your own?

Each of us will focus on different areas as more or less important to us, what is, however, clear is that each of these areas also has value and equal importance for people who have a learning disability. Unfortunately, however, for many people who have a learning disability achieving their aspirations within each of these areas can present additional challenges, as outlined in the next section.

Where we are now

One of the first areas of difficulty experienced by some people who have a learning disability is that of the struggle to convince their family to value them as an equal member and see them as someone they can rely on, for example, to help with organising the family party.

In addition, for many families the concept of mother/father son/daughter relationships can be overridden by the nature of the caring role (Grant 2005). An important aspect of the future training and development agenda is how to support families to return to their role as a parent rather than forcing them into a role as a carer, other than where this is an active choice made by the family.

The situation with friends can be equally complex. Many people who have a learning disability still find themselves in inequitable relationships. In addition, friendships may often be mediated by other people, such as parents, or may consist mostly of people paid to spend time with the individual rather than for the intrinsic value of simply being with the person. Whatever the reason, it is clear that while for some people friendships are now more meaningful, for a number of people this is still not happening (Butcher 2001). In support of this, the future workforce needs to be able to help people to assert themselves and to build bridges within their local communities (Butcher 2001).

Being healthy and working are often inextricably linked. For people who have a learning difficulty the relationship between employment and health is potentially more complex than for other people. Particularly because the number of people who have a learning disability who are employed is less than 10 per cent (Grove and Williams 2002), essentially leaving approximately 90 per cent of people who have a learning disability unemployed and facing the inherent health risks associated with this. This, combined with the known fact that people who have a learning disability can have significantly more health needs than other members of the population (Hatton et al. 2003), is concerning.

Home, as we have already stated, is crucially important to all of us. It was to this end that learning disability services have worked towards supporting people who have a learning disability to have tenancies. In many areas this has been highly successful, based on the belief that tenancies give people a degree of security that previously they did not have. The stark reality is that while this may be true to a certain degree, many tenancies are not legally binding and in some services people can still be asked to move out, for example, if their health needs change. As is well known, moving home can be the cause of significant stress as noted in the Holmes and Rahe Stress Adjustment Scale (Holmes and Rahe 1967).

Conversely, stress, in moderation, can be healthy. This is, however, if the stress can be acknowledged and managed. For people who have a learning disability this acknowledgement does not often exist, despite the number of stressful situations that can be imposed upon people, for example, the imposition of a new co-tenant or lack of meaningful activity during your week. When this is the case, stress can be damaging.

Leisure is inextricably intertwined with money, transport systems and support for many people who have a learning disability. Sometimes there are a number of examples where people find the physical access to services problematic, and the attitudes they encounter difficult and restrictive. Currently, therefore, people who have a learning difficulty can find accessing leisure opportunities difficult. This can then have spin-offs for people's health, and their overall quality of life. This area particularly demonstrates the importance of educating those people who work in the wider world outside learning disability services.

Having a history can establish our sense of who we are. For people who have a learning disability, often their history is lost among the recollections of people whom they no longer have any contact with, and professional records. If history is so important to us, how can we be so careless with the memories, experiences and recollections of other people? Currently the development of life books is an attempt to remedy this situation and the skills inherent in this approach are crucial for the future workforce. Also communication passports can help with this area (see Chapter 7 for more information). Most important though are friendships and relationships that help overcome the negative effect of changing support relationships.

Independence is a goal many of us aspire to, however, when we are exploring it for ourselves we feel that it is acceptable to be largely inter-dependent on a range of services and people. We also often describe it as doing what we want, when we want and with whom we want. Why, then, for people on the receiving end of services does independence take on a different meaning? It becomes a goal people have to work towards before they can access the community. It is something to test people against and label them if they are not independent. Developing the workforce to support people without testing them is crucial for the future.

In essence, what we have described so far are the things that are important to all of us, including people who have a learning disability. What we have also considered are the difficulties people who have a learning disability can experience in aspiring to an ordinary life and the implications for the work-force. The next section therefore will analyse the skills and knowledge required by the workforce in order to achieve these goals.

Values, knowledge and skills needed for the future workforce

In order to meet the needs of people who have a learning disability in the future we need to explore a number of different but interrelated aspects of the 'worker'. In particular, the support they deliver and the framework in which this is expressed. This means considering the values, the underpinning knowledge and the skills required by the worker (Department of Health 2005), whether these are actioned via a qualifications framework or not.

Value base

The issue of values is fundamentally important if people who have a learning disability are to be supported in the way they aspire to. It is equally an area that is not always given due regard with respect to professional training. The Learning Disability Award Framework (LDAF) now known as LDQ, as it currently stands, has attempted to integrate values into all aspects of the units it presents to inform the development of this part of the workforce.

The value base that those working with people who have a learning disability should be operating to is encapsulated primarily in the social model of disability (Finkelstein 1980; Oliver 1990). Some health professional courses have integrated this into the way they work with people as well as into social work courses. Others have, however, stayed very much within the framework that relates to their specific professional discipline. Reasons for this reluctance to embrace the social model of disability include statements such as 'the main focus of this course is achieving the professional integrity of those people who will be ascribed the professional title'. By that we mean that if you are training to be a nurse, then it is nursing theory that you should focus on as that is what makes you a nurse. Further rationale for not including the social model in the course is the belief that as the course is generic, it is difficult to include aspects that relate to one customer group only. The important principle here is that the social model of disability is not relevant to only one customer group. A good knowledge of this and associated models is relevant to all groups of people and is particularly important if we are to aspire to the ambitions of *Our Health, Our Care, Our Say* (Department of Health 2006). In addition, it will be crucial if we are to genuinely make the move to self-directed services and professionals are to be able to offer their gifts and expertise to people who use services.

It is, however, important to acknowledge that the social model of disability is an evolving model. This evolution has included a number of developments:

- the affirmation model (Swain and French 2000);
- the citizenship model (Duffy 2003).

The affirmation model

In this model the concepts and principles underpinning the social model of disability are developed to 'include' the person's impairment. This development was based upon criticism of the social model in which the disability people may have is not seen as being part of any of the difficulties they may experience in life. In essence, the social model acknowledges that all difficulties experienced by disabled people are the result of access issues or the attitudes of members of society. The affirmation model acknowledges the role that impairments or disabilities of people can have upon their ability to operate in life. In essence, it gives an additional responsibility to society to also mediate the person's impairment or disability (Swain and French 2000).

The citizenship model

This model forms the basis of the self-directed support model and as such is a direct response to those issues felt to be at fault within the professional gift model (Duffy 2003) (for more information, see Chapter 4). The citizenship model presumes that the person has an entitlement to the funding they require to live their life. Within this model the funding continues to be provided by the state and is used for an agreed purpose, usually to provide the support needed by the person to allow them to live their life. However, instead of the money going to a statutory organisation to be managed, it is given to the person to control. This simple transaction quickly and effectively changes the status of the person within their community. It places the person at the centre of their community with rights and responsibilities and economic power in the same way as many other people. Duffy (2003) identifies six keys to citizenship (see Chapter 4), knowledge and skills in each of these areas will be essential in the workforce of the future along with the ability to hand power back to people, individual budgets, support planning and brokerage. For any skill set to be delivered effectively, it is essential that they be informed by an appropriate knowledge base.

Underpinning knowledge

Underpinning knowledge effectively falls into four distinct categories:

- knowledge specific to the person being supported;
- generic knowledge useful to all people working within the sector;
- population, or service user group;
- profession-specific.

The knowledge specific to the individual is the most important level of knowledge required. All other levels should build on this in a way that is relevant to the person.

The generic knowledge base has been addressed in part in the section concerned with value base. However, additional areas for consideration include the following:

- communication skills, including accessible information;
- information technology, including assistive technology;
- citizenship;
- power and control;
- self-determination;
- quality monitoring;
- supported decision-making.

Population-specific knowledge would include areas such as the health needs of people who have a learning disability and intervention strategies specific to the profession. Community building may also form an essential part of the underpinning knowledge of a range of professions working in learning disabilities as would person centred approaches, skills and tools and person centred planning.

Activity 5.2

In addition to the knowledge areas identified above, what profession-specific knowledge do you feel would be important in a pre-qualifying course?

The profession-specific knowledge and its application are where the greatest differences would be between different curricula. By this it is meant those areas that differentiate between occupational therapy, medical professionals and social workers, etc. The fact these areas also need to be part of the curricula can create tensions regarding which issues are included as there is never sufficient time to include all aspects of what everyone believes should be included.

Skills

Skills that are viewed as being important to instil into the workforce in order to meet the needs of people are many. *Independence, Well-being and Choice* (Department of Health 2005) indicates the need for the workforce to be open, honest, warm, empathetic and respectful, while treating people with equity, being non-judgemental and challenging unfair discrimination. This reinforces the information from a regional project exploring the workforce needs of those individuals supporting people who have a learning disability. This work was completed in 2001 (Pickering and Thompson 2001) prior to some of the recent innovations in support. It does, however, give us a framework for considering the skills required by the workforce both now and in the future, see Box 5.1.

Box 5.1 Skills expected of people working with people who have a learning disability

---

- Communication – written, verbal, easy to understand, augmented communication.
- Empowerment, advocacy, assertiveness.
- Handing power back to people who have a learning difficulty.
- Managing and supporting people through transitions and life changes.
- Working in partnership, across agencies and across boundaries.
- Social inclusion, civil rights, choice, social networks or community building.
- Problem solving.
- Leisure and occupation, housing, employment, benefits.

(Pickering and Thompson 2001)

What people who have a learning disability want from the workforce

Having identified what the policy documents and the workforce in general think is important, it is essential to gain the view of people who have a learning disability on this question.

Activity 5.3

Talk to someone you know who has a learning disability about what skills they value in people who support them. How similar are these to what you think and what you thought the person would say?

Work with people who have a learning disability in one area indicated the wish for paid carers who were caring, helped the person to help others, listened and were helpful. People who looked after each other, were understanding and used their common sense. They also wanted individuals who they could have fun with, were helpful, worked as part of a team, respected them and were kind to them. They also felt it was important that people had good manners, were positive, had a good attitude and were pleasant. Finally, the person needed to be down to earth, happy, tell people when they have done a good job, look nice, offer choices, be trustworthy and help people to do the things they want to do (Dobson et al. 2002).

This information is reflected in the Trent Project (Ramcharan and Cutcliffe 2001) where service users identified the need for staff to be able to do the following:

- Communicate with the people they are working with. This includes the ability to use plain English and avoid the use of jargon, both in written and verbal formats.
- Effectively involve service users in service development and delivery, e.g. meetings, reviews, assessment, service planning and evaluation and recruitment of staff.
- Empower service users and enable them to take control of their own lives.
- Maintain confidentiality in respect of any conversations and discussions that take place.
- Give appropriate and understandable information so that service users can make good choices.

Souza (2006) identifies the need for support staff to help people to understand their own health, and help develop a meaningful life in order to give the person a reason to be healthy and an understanding of sexual health, to name but a few.

At the same time as knowing what they do want from their support, people using services are also clear about what they do not want. The following list was developed as a consequence of a study on recruitment that was undertaken in Bradford. In this work people using services stated very clearly that they did not want support from people who:

- only think about themselves;
- make fun behind the person's back;
- are ignorant;
- think they are better than the person they support and treat them like a kid/baby;
- interrupt;
- tell people they support to be quiet;
- use big words;
- are bossy;
- tell people what to do all the time;
- lose their rag;
- make/tell people to do things they do not want to do;
- swear;
- shout;
- are nasty;
- bite people's head off;

- name call;
- talk in front of the person as if they are not there.

Implications for education

Analysis of this information and the literature/policy poses particular challenges to people developing curricula. The challenge is how to take the essential list of skills, and ensure the person has the relevant underpinning knowledge base, the correct values and pulls all these aspects together to inform the correct delivery of the support/intervention in a way that is positive for the person with a learning disability and those around them. By that it is meant that the support is highly person centred and the person is placed at the centre of their life, not just the centre of the intervention. A particular challenge is to take the values, knowledge and skills identified here and to intertwine them into a professional curricula in such a way that supports the achievement of an ordinary life and citizenship.

For example, this means not just delivering communication skills training in the way we always have but in a way that supports the professional to, for example, better identify what is important to the person about their family and how to relate to them, what is important to the person about their community and how they wish to interact with members of their community or what stressors a person experiences and what they wish to do in relation to each one. All of the above can be achieved to greater or lesser degrees and in part or by all of the workforce. One key strategy for achieving this is to include person centred thinking skills and person centred tools in all curricula as well as person centred planning. The level to which this is achieved, however, is dependent upon the parts of the workforce that are targeted for action. These are explored in the next section.

Future options for training and developing the workforce

The fact that both the aspirations of people and policy are indicating such fundamental changes to the way individuals are supported within our society when they are ill, disabled or in need of assistance, indicates the need to radically rethink the way we prepare the workforce. Currently we have a system that includes National Vocational Qualifications, i.e. competency-based training. In England this is underpinned by the Learning Disability Awards Framework, which at the time of writing is a vocationally-related qualification. This award is supported within *Valuing People* and is seen as a model of good practice within Skills for Care, the Sector Skills Council.

Paralleling this approach are a range of professional qualifications, some of which are learning disability-specific. The learning disability-specific qualifications currently include the Registered Nurse in Learning Disabilities qualification. The majority of the other professional qualifications are generic at the pre-qualifying level with specialist qualifications as the person progresses through their career. A good example of this would be Psychiatry. While this is the current model of workforce that we have, the question needs to be asked about whether this is the most appropriate model for the future.

Possibly the professions would argue it is. This then raises the question, is this the best group of people to make this decision? If the answer is no, then who can make the decision? People who have a learning difficulty could be asked. Their typical responses, however, are likely to be that they do not care what profession it is as long as their needs are met appropriately. People who have a learning disability are able to articulate what is important but not how this relates to professional structures and processes in workforce development.

Potentially the Sector Skills Councils (Matley and Addis 2002) could do this in partnership with the Care Services Improvement Partnership (CSIP). However, the professions are predominantly the domain of Skills for Health while the lead in learning disabilities workforce development is with Skills for Care. This may or may not prove problematic. However, one structure that is currently emerging in England is a group where these two organisations, the Valuing People Support Team, the Department of Health and others, meet together to explore the workforce needs of the learning disability sector. Perhaps here is the place for some more strategic thinking, and negotiating further partnerships that may need to exist at a strategic level. This group would, however, need to explore a range of options if they were to tackle the workforce agenda in such a fundamental way (see Table 5.1).

A further option exists that should be run in parallel to those described above, that is to increase the capacity of communities to accept people who are different, such as people who have a learning disability. This would effectively need to become a key focus of the work of a number of people, both people working directly with people who have a learning disability and those specialist professionals such as community nurses.

Activity 5.4

Describe the skills you think are important in building community capacity.

Working with communities would require skills and knowledge in the following areas (O'Brien and O'Brien 1991):

- community connecting;
- citizenship;
- developing friendships and relationships;

Table 5.1 Agenda options

Option	Advantages	Disadvantages
do nothing	• status quo maintained	• growing expectations remain unmet • tension continues to exist about what people want and how to get it • professionals unable to offer their full range of gifts to people
do nothing with professional groups and focus on the vocational workforce	• manageable as changes would be via NVQ and VRQ routes • challenge professionals to rethink their contributions	• professional groups still operating from same premise • tensions continue to exist
changes to vocational workforce and to continuing professional development agenda	• impacts on greater number of people therefore greater outcomes • easier than changing pre-qualifying courses	• people influenced by the change are not the full range of people who need to be affected • risk there is no critical mass in the workplace to influence change
changes to vocational workforce and to pre-qualifying courses within the area of vulnerable adults	• impacts on all of the immediate workforce • includes people outside of learning disability services who may come into contact with people who have a learning disability • mainstreams some of the learning disability agendas	• greater number of stakeholders to influence • more curricula restrictions to deal with • more professional body issues to address
different approach to training people who work with people who have a learning disability	• the workforce would more readily reflect the needs of the people it serves	• years of history to undo • professional body issue to address • professional cultures to work with • many people will not want this to happen due to their professional identity and what they believe about their profession and its importance

- sustaining and ending relationships;
- community mapping;
- social networks;
- problem solving;
- conflict resolution;
- developing partnerships.

In summary, to truly meet the needs of people who have a learning disability in the future, we need to think creatively and strategically about the changes that need to be made to the current systems and structures of workforce development. This includes the structures supporting professional education across welfare services. Much of this change cannot be achieved by individuals developing and delivering qualifications, only by major strategic change. So what can individuals do? Individuals can think about the implications of the things discussed so far in this chapter and embrace them for the value and the difference they will make to people who have a learning disability rather than reject them because they are too difficult. They can also work proactively to support any proposals that may arise in the future in order to meet the challenges of the next 20 years. But most importantly you can consider some of the smaller changes that you can effect within the courses you deliver. These are outlined in the next section.

Next steps

A simple and achievable first step would be to consider how current education programmes both for professionals at pre- and post-qualifying levels as well as the vocationally qualified workforce, could become more person centred. An additional step would be to look at how the social model of disability, the affirmation model, the citizenship model and the values ensconced in contemporary policy could become an integral part of all programmes. Exploration of each of the above potential changes has both a theoretical and practice-focused application.

Theory

The starting point within any application of person centredness and the different models, outlined above, has to be the clear acknowledgement that all professional courses are structured differently. This therefore means that some of the first steps outlined in this chapter will be easier to include in some curricula than others. But as has been said many times before, we do not achieve the things that are important without much effort. Most professional education within welfare services is now commissioned via the Strategic

Health Authorities. The exception to this is social work and the medical professions.

Integrating person centredness into the different courses can occur on a number of different levels. The first level of integration should be in relation to values and attitudes. Courses that already include modules or content in relation to this area may find this an obvious place to include the relevant information. It is essential that these include the social model of disability, the affirmation model and citizenship. Delivery of this information should allow people to explore their values and beliefs, be challenged safely on these issues and leave the session feeling safe while having rethought some of their values and beliefs in a more person centred way. In essence, these explorations should take place in a supportive, thinking environment (Kline 2004). Fundamental to this will be individuals' understanding of the difference between the professional gift model and the citizenship model. This will give people the basis for future work. It provides a way to challenge professionals, services and the way they themselves affect other people. Essentially, it should form the basis of developing thoughtful, empowered professionals who will translate this into all their actions and subsequently empower the people on the receiving end of support.

Having established the appropriate value base, it is essential to consider the person centred approaches, skills and tools that can be incorporated into the curricula. These may fall naturally into sessions on assessment, or planning care, transitions and communication. Assessment may include discussions on what works well and what is not working as a way of gathering data, also using MAP and PATH to identify people's dreams and aspirations will be appropriate for some professionals. In communication sessions consideration of areas such as communication maps could prove useful, or learning logs. Other tools that are important to include in the curricula are '4 plus 1' questions, communication dictionaries, important to and important for, the doughnut, or staff matching tools to name a few (for more detail on each of these, see Chapters 3 and 7). At this stage it is important that we are still embedding the approaches within the person prior to then considering the implications and opportunities to work with professionals in relation to person centred planning.

Incorporating person centred planning training in professional courses requires creativity and a capacity to think differently. One place this may happen is at the end of a pre-qualifying course or immediately afterwards. This way it builds upon the previous learning and experience in order to maximise outputs. If this is not achievable, then it should still be possible to incorporate an understanding of person centred planning in pre-qualifying curricula. This can be done in a variety of contexts, working with families, particularly picking up on families leading planning and family essential lifestyle plans, advocacy modules or sessions, focusing upon people leading their own plans. Modules or sessions addressing health issues and the health needs of the population could consider not only Health Action Plans (Department of Health 2002) but also person centred planning and how these two planning approaches can be integrated (for more information, see Chapter 6).

Having explored some of the possible ways of including person centred-ness and associated values into a range of curricula, the other crucial aspect that requires consideration is how to make practice more person centred.

Practice

Practice is typically delivered through a placement approach. This is the way most courses have always been organised. Consequently most people struggle to conceptualise any other way to deliver practice experience. At the same time we are surrounded by people who are critical of the quality of newly qualified staff, professionals who do not feel fit to practise or people who are struggling to deliver curricula because of the constraints of practice. Essentially, then, the current system has many concerns that can be levelled at it, leaving ample opportunity to consider more creative solutions. If at the same time we could also deliver a more person centred approach that demonstrates the applicability of the models we have referred to, then that has to be a positive option.

While such a model may feel a long way away, we believe that one already does exist. This approach is typically referred to in the earlier literature as client allocation or client attachment (Renouf 1990), it has, however, more recently been renamed individual-led practice (Thompson and Cobb 2005).

Individual-led practice

In this approach students do not have placements, they undertake practice experience. This typically means students work with between three and five people at any one time. These people should be living and working in different areas and should all have different needs. The aim of this is to ensure the student has the widest possible experience available. Because each student works with the individual on a specific area of need that is real to them and relevant to the student's learning, it allows the students to operate from a more person centred perspective. This is particularly as individual practice is not driven by end points to practise experiences or routines that typically exist in practice settings. Within this role they may find themselves initiating, co-ordinating, contributing or safeguarding a person centred plan (for more information, see Chapter 2). Alternatively they may find themselves using some of the person centred approaches identified in Chapters 3 and 7.

Fundamental to the success of this approach is the student's ability to identify the skills they still need to develop, and the experiences they still need to have. Because they are not given an end point to their involvement with a person (other than the end of the course), the student is able to follow any piece of work through from initiation or referral through planning and implementation to completion or disengagement. Experience indicates that following through this process allows the student to understand the interrelationship between each aspect of the process much more effectively than those students who practise each step with a different person.

With this approach people who are receiving support also gain control over the situation. The student has to gain the person's initial permission for any work they may do, in addition to gaining ongoing support. Examples have occurred where people who have a learning disability have either voted with their feet, by not being at home when a student visits or disengaging from the student. In such situations students can be left feeling extremely uncomfortable, and rejected. As part of the process of individual-led practice the student needs to reflect on the situation. This level of control for the person who has a learning disability often does not exist in a placement model. In this context the student will often continue to be placed in the environment even if they are not expected to work with the person directly. In models where the service user is able to demonstrate that level of control the students have to seriously rethink the power balance.

When working within a system that allows the student to work flexibly a number of other aspects support the person centredness and citizenship agenda. These include the opportunity to meet the needs of individuals in whatever setting the person is working with them, either at home, in day services or employment settings. It also supports the student working in whichever of these environments is appropriate rather than confining them to the placement identified on an allocations sheet (Thompson and Cobb 2005). In addition, this approach allows the student to support people in areas that the person feels is important, not what the professional feels is necessary.

One note of caution in this approach to practice, however, has to be that the supervisory structure that needs to be placed around individual-led practice must be rigorous, timely and focused on practice, evidence and accountability. As well as demanding a high level of supervision, this approach also demands that supervision is person centred. Some of the tools identified in Chapter 3 could prove useful in this context. Additional complexities to consider include the significant shift in thinking that is required to move the curriculum from one that is placement-led to one that is led by choice, flexibility and research or evidence-based practice. Within such a flexible approach where students cannot be guaranteed that they will have been taught all they need to know about a particular group of people or a label, before they commence working with a person they need to build appropriate research time into their working week. Thus, a student and ultimately a professional develops who appreciates the need to research their interventions rather than one who searches for the justification for their actions after the event in order to meet a specific course requirement.

While a more person centred approach to teaching and to practice is an excellent first step to take towards the changing demands on the workforce, it is also important to consider the implications of introducing a worker into a workforce that has not yet had the chance to explore the issues that the individual has considered. The impact of this can lead to personal frustration and in some instances failure. This is particularly true as conformity to the established norm can be powerful in services working to support individuals. Failure is often due to the number of people espousing 'new ways of working' often being in the minority. What is therefore helpful is a critical mass of people wanting to achieve the same goal. This can be helped through the provision of continuing professional development opportunities for most people.

Continuing professional development and person centredness

Essentially this can be addressed by including all aspects of the proposals for pre-qualifying courses but also by developing opportunities for people to undertake a number of post-qualifying courses/modules. These modules can include the value base underpinning person centred planning and approaches, person centred planning, facilitator training, person centred reviews and support planning and individualised budgets.

Ideally, each of these modules or learning experiences should be delivered from a multi-professional perspective and should include people who have a learning disability, social care and health care workers, people from the independent sector and family carers. Some areas have proved more successful than others in gaining this mix of people participating on course. Only by doing this will we move closer to the goals in policy documents (Department of Health 2001, 2006: Scottish Executive 2000) and more effectively meet the aspirations of people.

Conclusion

What is clear from both this chapter and the rest of this book is that we are in a time of major change. The potential to finally achieve all the important things that people who have a learning disability want is here and now. This means that the expectations on both the professionally and vocationally qualified workforce will change. In order to meet these changes we need to address a number of key issues identified within this chapter. These changes will be more effective, the more radical the changes. It is down to the workforce and those who train and educate these individuals to embrace these changes.

Some of the major changes, if they are to happen, will take many years, the next steps have to be the place to start, in order to make some immediate differences for people who have a learning disability.

References

Acheson, D. (1998) *Independent Inquiry into Inequalities in Health*. London: Department of Health.

Atkinson, D. (2005) Narrative and people with learning disabilities, in G. Grant, P. Goward, M. Richardson and P. Ramcharan *Learning Disability: A Life Cycle Approach to Valuing People*. Maidenhead: Open University Press.

Butcher, A. (2001) Working with communities, in J. Thompson and S. Pickering (eds) *Meeting the Health Needs of People Who Have a Learning Disability*. Edinburgh: Bailliere Tindall.

Department of Health (2001) *Valuing People: A New Strategy for Learning Disability for the 21st Century*. London: Department of Health.

Department of Health (2002) *Action for Health, Health Action Planning and Health Facilitation: Good Practice Guidance on Implementation for Learning Disability Partnership Boards*. London: HMSO.

Department of Health (2005) *Independence, Well-being and Choice: Our Vision for the Future of Social Care for Adults in England*. London: Department of Health.

Department of Health (2006) *Our Health, Our Care, Our Say*. London, HMSO. The Stationery Office.

Dobson, S., Upadhyaya, S. and Stanley, B. (2002) Using an interdisciplinary approach to training to develop the quality of communication with adults with profound learning disabilities by care staff; *International Journal of Language and Communication Disorders*, 37(1): 1–57.

Duffy, S. (2003) *Keys to Citizenship: A Guide to Getting Good Support Services for People with Learning Difficulties*. Birkenhead: Paradigm.

Finkelstein, V. (1980) *Attitudes and Disabled People*. New York: World Rehabilitation Fund.

Grant, G. (2005) Experiences of family care, in G. Grant, P. Goward, M. Richardson and P. Ramcharan *Learning Disability: A Life Cycle Approach to Valuing People*. Maidenhead: Open University Press.

Grove, B. and Williams, B. (2002) Employment framework, available at: http://www.valuingpeople.gov.uk/documents/EmploymentMainDocument.pdf accessed 27 June 2006.

Hatton, C., Elliott, J. and Emerson, E. (2003) Key highlights of research evidence on the health of people with learning disabilities, available at: http://www.valuingpeople.gov.uk/documents/HealthKeyHighlights.pdf accessed 27 June 2006.

Hewitt, H. (2006) *Life Story Books for People with Learning Disabilities: A Practical Guide*. Kidderminster: BILD Publications.

Holmes, T.H. and Rahe, R.H. (1967) The social readjustment rating scale, *Journal Psychosom Res.* 2: 213–18.

Kline, N. (2004) *Time to Think: Listening to Ignite the Human Mind*. New York: Basic Books.

Matley, H. and Addis, M. (2002) Competence-based training, vocational qualifications and learning targets: some lessons for the learning and skills council, *Education and Training*, 44(6): 250–60.

O'Brien, J. and O'Brien, C.L. (1991) *Members of Each Other*. Toronto: Inclusion Press.

Oliver, M. (1990) *The Politics of Disablement*. London: Macmillan.

Pickering, S. and Thompson, J. (2001) *Meeting the Health Needs of People Who Have a Learning Disability*. London: Elsevier.

Ramcharan, P. and Cutcliffe, J.R. (2001) Judging the ethics of qualitative research: considering the 'ethics as process' model, *Health and Social Care in the Community*, 9(6): 358–66.

Renouf, C. (1990) Client allocation, paper presented at English National Board for Nursing Midwifery and Health Visiting National Conference, 23–26 July, Ripon.

Rolph, S., Atkinson, D., Nind, M. and Welshman, J. (2005) *Witness to Change*. Kidderminster: BILD Publications.

Scottish Executive (2000) *The Same as You? A Review of Services for People with Learning Disabilities*, Edinburgh: Scottish Executive.

Selye, H. (1956) General adaptation syndrome, in H. Selye (1974) *Stress without Distress*. London: Hodder and Stoughton.

Souza, A. (2006) Being well, my well being, in S. Pickering and J. Thompson (eds) *Meeting the Health Needs of People Who Have a Learning Disability*. London: Elsevier.

Swain, J. and French, S. (2000) Towards an affirmation model of disability, *Disability & Society*, 15(4): 569–82.

Thompson, J. and Cobb, J. (2005) Person centred approaches to education, *RCN Learning Disability Practice*, 7(5): 12–15.

Thompson, J. and Westwood, L. (2007) What is important to you? *Association of Practitioners in Learning Disability*, 23(3): 8–14.

Useful resources

Helen Sanderson Associates
www.helensandersonassociates.co.uk

in Control
www.in-control.org.uk

6 Person centred approaches to meeting the health needs of people who have a learning disability

Jeanette Thompson with Janet Cobb

Key issues

- Health action planning
- Person centred planning
- Person centred thinking skills and tools
- Introducing, contributing, safeguarding and integrating person centred planning and health action planning

Introduction

It is now well acknowledged that people who have a learning disability have higher health needs than other members of the general population. This picture is particularly complicated by the number of associated health needs of many people who have a learning disability, this combination of health need is typically referred to as co-morbidity. In addition, Moss and Turner (1995) state that the health of the population of people who have a learning disability changes over time, as it does for the remainder of the population. This is seen to be the result of the interface between ageing and morbidity and mortality patterns. For the general population this selectivity becomes more noticeable in later life, but for people who have a learning disability it can have a marked effect throughout life. It is for these reasons that attention to the health of people who have a learning disability is crucially important.

Valuing People (Department of Health 2001) set a clear direction for meeting the health needs of people who have a learning disability as well as for other areas of their lives. This vision, underpinned by a full belief in citizenship for people who have a learning disability, was to achieve this through a particular focus on rights, choice, independence and inclusion. In *Valuing People* a number of key areas were identified for services to work on; these included leading a fulfilling life and as already stated, being healthy. Each of these areas had key approaches that were to be used to support achieving the targets set out in the White Paper. For fulfilling lives, person centred planning was to be the approach of choice, and for health and well-being a concept called health action planning (HAP) was introduced. In *Valuing People* and subsequent guidance, key messages were presented about the need to integrate both these approaches.

Moving on from *Valuing People*, almost as an evolution of the goals and aims within this policy document, many areas are now actively working towards an approach called self-directed support. Fundamental to this way of supporting people is the concept of citizenship and rights. In particular, it articulates a move from the professional gift model to one of citizenship (see Chapter 4 for a discussion of these different approaches). In essence, therefore, when thinking about the health needs of people who have a learning disability, it is important to think about a number of underlying principles. These include, the need to integrate person centred planning (PCP) and health action planning as one approach, how to better use person centred thinking, person centred planning and person centred approaches to develop health action plans on those occasions they cannot be integrated. Lastly, how we will meet the health needs of people who have a learning disability when they are in control of their lives and making decisions about their lives. Before considering each of these key issues, it is important to consider the current situation.

Consideration of what is happening around the country at the time of writing indicates a highly variable position in relation to the identified goal of one plan (Department of Health 2001). What is known is that many people have health action plans. Equally we have many people with person centred plans, some of which address health issues as a natural part of the person centred planning process. However, these are not in sufficient numbers to achieve the goal of one plan and often are not part of a deliberate and structured attempt to integrate the two approaches.

Activity 6.1

What issues help and what makes it difficult to integrate health action plans within person centred plans?

People find this difficult for a variety of reasons, these include the following:

- the different priority groups identified in *Valuing People* for both HAP and PCP;
- resources;
- timing;
- ownership;
- the developments within person centred planning and the move towards person centred practice.

Person centred planning was given clear *priority groups* to work with in *Valuing People*. These included older people, people in transition, people on hospital campuses and in long-stay hospital settings, people with older carers and those whose day services were being changed. These target groups were all identified for good reason. However, what this meant was that the resources available in person centred planning were often busy focusing on these priorities and therefore not able to address additional work such as interfacing person centred planning and health action planning. At the same time many people working within health settings did not always have the opportunity to address this issue, particularly as much of their time was spent working with primary care to address the issues of mainstreaming the responsibility to meet the health needs of the learning disability population.

Resources are also an important factor impacting on the difficulties experienced in integrating health action plans and person centred plans. This includes the skill set of the workforce, in relation to values, approaches, knowledge, skills, tools and planning. In addition, it includes the availability of resources when they are needed.

Timing is also an issue, health action plans can be something that is required with immediate effect, depending on the person's circumstances. Quite often person centred plans are developed over a longer period of time. The challenge to health professionals, if we are to integrate health within person centred planning approaches, is to identify how this can be achieved. This may mean thinking creatively about different ways to record and action health issues with the person and within their plan.

Ownership has also proved challenging at different points in time. Lengthy discussions have taken place in some parts of the country about who should complete health action plans and how this should be done. Different solutions have included person centred planning facilitators completing health action plans often around lifestyle issues, or health professionals being part of the person centred planning team. Some areas have dealt with the issue of ownership by bringing together health facilitators and person centred planning co-ordinators in order to work through approaches to health action planning.

Whichever approach has been used, questions still arise in some parts of the country about how to achieve the goal of integrated person centred plans and health action plans. Fundamental to this debate and a possible way to help solve the current difficulty is the principle that the plan should be owned by the person. When an individual has a person centred plan, this is clearly the case, with a separate health action plan this should also be the case, however, it can on occasions become the professional's document, with all the problems inherent with this. If we are able to move to a position where the person owns the health action plan, then the issue of integrating person centred plans and health action plans becomes easier to achieve and the choice of the individual.

Finally, the recent *changes in person centred planning* have also added to the complexity of the situation. By this we are referring to the significant developments within this community of practice. Developments such as families leading planning, person centred reviews, person centred approaches and the associated skills and tools (for more detail on these, see Chapters 2, 3, 7, 10 and 11).

None of these issues or developments are problematic in themselves and many have been a natural progression of person centred planning. However, from the perspective of trying to achieve integrated person centred plans and health action plans, it is easy to see why for many people it simply became too difficult.

From the information above we can clearly see it can be difficult to ensure health needs and health action plans are integrated into a person centred plan. However, if we are to achieve the important goal of people not having too many different influences in their lives, and ensuring those that they do have are within the person's control, then it is important to integrate questions relating to health and health action plans into person centred plans. Some person centred planning tools already include questions relating to health needs, for example, Personal Futures Planning. In these circumstances it is sensible to continue with the integrated approach. In continuing to develop this approach to meeting the health needs of a person, the role of the professional becomes one of either safeguarding or contributing to the process. These and other professional roles are considered later in the chapter.

If the planning process is like PATH, however, then health may not come up as an issue and in these instances a separate plan could prove necessary. This should, however, be the individual's decision. Other instances where a separate plan may be useful is when the person's health needs are so complex that they cannot be addressed sufficiently within the person centred plan. A natural extension from this, if the health action plan is developed in a person centred way and the person does not have a person centred plan, then this may be seen as the first step towards collecting person centred information which could ultimately grow into a person centred plan for the person. This would be one way of addressing the tensions created by the priority groups and the timing issue.

For people who fall into the category of having a separate health action plan, it is therefore very important to consider how we can develop that plan using person centred approaches, tools and skills. The starting point for this is the guidance in *Valuing People*, which indicated that the plan belongs to the person, is about the aspects of their health that the person (not necessarily the professional) finds important and that the health action plan should be in a format that makes sense to the person.

Person centred health action plans

A great deal of work has taken place in this area with a range of different tools being made available to help people manage their health. These range from health passports, hospital books and health checks, health records, through to larger publications which address the whole process of developing a health action plan. While each of these focuses on the person and places them at the centre of the intervention relating to their health or health need, it is rare that any of these approaches utilises the skills and tools inherent within person centred planning to ensure that we are being truly person centred in how we develop health action plans. This next section will consider a range of these tools, many of which are described in detail in other chapters within this book. In this chapter we will be looking at their value in relation to meeting the health needs of someone who has a learning disability and developing their health action plan where relevant. The tools, approaches and skills we will be exploring include:

- essential lifestyle planning;
- personal futures planning;
- person centred reviews;
- person centred thinking tools;
- accessible information (total communication).

Essential lifestyle planning

Essential lifestyle planning was developed as part of the planning and resettlement of people leaving long-stay institutions in the USA (Smull and Harrison 1992). These approaches allow us to explore the details of how a person wishes to be supported on a daily basis. It is for this reason that the approaches within essential lifestyle planning can work particularly well for people's health needs. Within the overall approach in essential lifestyle planning a key question that is integral to any planning process is 'What do you need to stay healthy and safe?' An essential lifestyle plan fundamentally describes what is important to someone and what is important for them to stay healthy and safe. This would typically address the person's health in a range of areas, for example:

- teeth and gums;
- staying fit and active/mobility;
- continence;
- eyesight;
- hearing;
- healthy eating;
- medicines;
- health checks;
- emotional well-being;
- supporting sexual health and relationships.

Each of the areas above that are of relevance to the individual can be explored using a key set of questions. These are:

- What support does the person need?
- From the person's perspective, what does good support look like?
- From the person's perspective, what does bad support look like?
- What does this mean we/the person need to do?

Activity 6.2

Think about a person who you are working with to develop a health action plan. With each area of their plan, think about the questions listed above. What information does that give you about how the person should be supported?

As you might expect, there will be a range of responses to this question. What might help to judge how you may develop an individual's health action plan with them can be seen in Maggie's health action plan (Table 6.1). This was developed using the essential lifestyles approach to planning and is just one part of a much more extensive document. The rest of this document can be found at www.helensandersonassociates.co.uk

Maggie has depression which she calls 'not well' which is cyclic and seems to be more severe at the time of her menstrual cycle. She is currently taking Seroxate which is working very well.

You know Maggie is becoming unwell:

- when she does not want to get up in the morning;
- when she has a poor appetite;
- when she does not want to go to work;
- when she wants to spend the day in her bedroom away from the others;
- when she tries to harm herself – by scratching her legs and feet.

Table 6.1 Maggie's health action plan

Good support when Maggie is 'not well'	Bad support when Maggie is 'not well'
Knowing her well and spotting the signs that Maggie isn't well	Being supported by people she does not know or like is a definite no-no!
An extra hour in bed and then offering a warm bubble bath – don't rush or be confrontational with her	People forcing her to do things she doesn't want to do or being confrontational with her
Helping her more with dressing	Asking her loads of questions
Watching the TV in her bedroom and doing some artwork	Being in the middle of a lot of hustle and bustle
Checking that she is OK at regular intervals (although not in an obtrusive way)	Not checking that she is OK
	Trying to physically stop her from harming herself – better to distract Maggie into her artwork, watching TV or going for a walk

Preventing Maggie harming herself
If she does harm herself, stay with her, doing some art and watching TV with her, without bombarding her with questions about it
Sometimes going out for a walk works really well
Make sure she is offered choices of foods which she really likes (see Most, Second and Third in Importance)
She also will ask for cups of tea throughout the day
Make sure her environment is peaceful and quiet
Having a chat with Maggie about her day sometimes helps
Maggie also needs to see her doctor every two days when she feels like this. Maggie finds a lot of comfort from seeing her doctor when she feels like this
Keep a record of how she is feeling to share with the doctor

Therefore what works best in supporting Maggie is to:

- Make sure that the people supporting her are people she knows well and likes.
- If she does not want to get up, come back in an hour and run her a nice bath with loads of bubbles.
- Do not rush her or be confrontational with her.

- Help her more with dressing.
- Check she is OK every hour (unobtrusively) to make sure she is safe.
- Knowing Maggie is more content when in her bedroom watching TV and doing her artwork.
- If she is upset and you think she might harm herself, stay with her, having chats, watching telly.
- Do not bombard her with questions about how she is feeling.
- Offering to go out for a walk (if the weather's nice) also sometimes takes her mind off it.

Personal futures planning

In personal futures planning, there is a 'map' that focuses on health. It is split into two sections:

1   conditions that lead to good health;
2   conditions that lead to poor health.

The same areas identified in essential lifestyle planning can be used in personal futures planning, for example, if the area was: 'to keep my teeth and gums healthy', then the personal futures planning would show:

1   conditions that lead to me having good oral health care;
2   conditions that lead to me having poor oral health care.

Person centred reviews

Person centred reviews started their life in schools as part of a process to try and improve the young person's and their family's experience of their school reviews. The very nature of the existing system combined with the overly professionalised approach to most of these reviews meant that the whole concept of person centred reviews had to operate within some very tight parameters. Person centred reviews can therefore, when necessary, operate within a tight timescale. They use many of the key questions relating to person centred approaches, starting with 'What do we like and admire about a person?' This is a crucially important question that in the world of the health professional can be lost, primarily because the professional tends to be called in to deal with a problematic issue, for example, behaviour, mobility or sexuality. To include this in the automatic way that any professional works would significantly shift the balance of how the person is perceived and consequently how professionals work with individuals to keep them at the centre of their lives rather than just at the centre of their professional intervention.

Subsequent questions include 'What is working well for the person?' and 'What is not working for the person?' To ask these two questions in the context of an individual's health could result in some significant information being aired that will help with the development of a person centred health action plan.

Activity 6.3

When you are developing a health action plan with an individual, how much do you base your work on the principles of what works and does not work for the person to inform what is included in the plan?

An analysis of John's plan (Table 6.2) can indicate the level of detail needed if health action plans are to become person centred. Those people reading the 'what does not work' for John and finding reasons why this cannot happen where they work are beginning to identify how the constraints of some environments mean we are not as person centred as we need to be. In these instances we need to work much harder to make our work with people, person centred.

Table 6.2 John's health action plan

Good support: when John's chest is bad he needs	Bad support: when John's chest is bad would look like this
• To see a doctor who will usually prescribe liquid antibiotics • To be positioned in as upright a position as possible for John to be comfortable to help him breathe more easily • Lots of contact with the people supporting John to reassure him he is OK • To be offered drinks every hour, John has a small beaker of warm tea with one sugar or Vimto/Blackcurrant cordial (tepid) • The tisAnn under John's chin to be changed regularly so his jumper/neck does not become wet due to dribbling • To change position every 30 minutes (options repositioning are in John's physio plan)	• Being supported into his standing frame to assist in the removal of chest secretions if he is feeling poorly • Lying flat • Going out in wet and windy weather • Being left alone • Not being offered drinks • Not being spoken to and reassured by those supporting him • Spending too long (more than 30 minutes) in his wheelchair • Clothes becoming wet due to dribbling • People supporting John who do not know him well, his inability to express pain means that those around him must know how he communicates through facial expression • Being supported to eat or drink in a poor position which could cause food inhalation

(This is one small part of John's plan, the rest can be found at www.helensandersonassociates.co.uk.)

A further question in person centred reviews that can be useful is asking the individual 'What is important for the future?' Answers to this question could include, for example, a person wanting to lose weight in order to look good on the beach when they go on holiday the following year. Including ways to address this in the person's health action plan would very clearly need to link to the responses to the what works and what does not work questions. Another significant question in the person centred reviews framework is 'What is needed to keep the person healthy and safe?' This question is particularly important as it can be an opportunity to address issues that people around the individual feel are important but have not been identified by the person themselves. The final question within person centred reviews focuses on the questions that are important to all in the room that have not yet been answered – 'Questions to answer' – it is a mop-up question that ensures anything that has not been covered throughout the process is now raised. Again this could be hugely useful in the context of a person's health, it also provides a safety net for professionals who may not in the first instance have confidence in person centred approaches.

Person centred thinking tools

Much has been written in this book about person centred thinking skills and person centred thinking tools. This section will consider some of the tools described in Chapters 4 and 7, and how they can usefully contribute to meeting a person's health needs and the development of a health action plan. The tools we will consider include:

- important to and important for;
- doughnut;
- working/not working;
- 4 plus 1 questions;
- communication charts;
- learning logs;
- decision-making agreement.

Important to and important for

This approach to identifying important information in relation to an individual's health can be quite challenging. This is particularly linked to the fact that in most instances professionals tend to focus on what is 'important for' a person. Typical examples of what may fall within the category of what is 'important for' a person include taking their medication, managing their epilepsy or managing their behaviour, while what is 'important to' refers to what matters to the person and what matters now.

Identifying what is 'important to' a person in relation to their health is crucially important if we are to both help people improve their health in a sustainable way and also if we are going to operate in partnership with people in the new world that will be determined through self-directed support. Equally important within this is the need to balance what is 'important to' with what is 'important for' the person. This is so that the person can meet their health needs in a way that includes what is important to them at the same time as ensuring they are not being left vulnerable or at risk.

Sharon is a young woman who is severely obese. She has been told by her GP that she needs to lose weight. This is important for her. Sharon, however, really likes chocolate and eats at least one bar of chocolate each day. The team supporting her have referred her to a dietician who has put her on a strict diet in which she is not allowed any chocolate at all throughout the week. This particular approach very clearly addressed the issue of what is *important for* Sharon, i.e. to lose weight, it did not, however, address what is *important to* her. What is really important here is to balance what is *important to* and *important for* in order to produce a workable and sustainable solution to the problem. Different solutions could have included, supporting Sharon to have small amounts of chocolate each day, and doing more exercise to balance this, or a less frequent intake of chocolate.

The doughnut

The doughnut can be used by staff to identify what their core responsibilities are, in this instance, in relation to the person's health needs. This forms the central core of the doughnut. Around this we are also able to explore the areas in which creativity and judgement can be utilised and what is not the responsibility of a paid professional. One team working with a gentleman who was sleeping with a couple who lived near him used this approach in a multi-professional meeting to identify what the team's responsibilities were. In relation to their core responsibilities they agreed they needed to make sure he understood the nature of consensual sex, what constitutes an abusive relationship, issues around sexually transmitted diseases, to refer him into the adult protection process and to continue to give him the opportunity to talk to them and to change his mind about continuing in the relationship.

Creativity and judgement they felt informed the way they managed their discussions with him, the way in which they presented information about the different issues to him and the continued involvement of members of the team in the hope that he might choose to change the relationship he had with this couple. The not our paid responsibility part was very clearly about the fact that he was a consenting adult who understood what he was consenting to, got some feeling of value and human warmth from the relationship and he enjoyed the sex. As he had the capacity to consent to the relationship and the team had documented their efforts and their discussions around this issue, they agreed it was not the team's responsibility to stop the relationship. What they needed to focus on was keeping him as safe as possible within it.

Working/not working

This is the same as the questions about what is working and not working within person centred reviews. Within the context of health needs and health action planning it can be used very effectively to help someone to manage their behaviour as well as other areas, such as how to support someone to manage their diabetes or epilepsy. When a person has identified what is working for them in managing their health, then the focus is to work out how to continue with these successes. With respect of areas that are not working, then we need to consider what needs to change to ensure success for the individual.

4 plus 1 questions

Once again, these questions are designed to help us work out what we need to do with and for a person that works from their perspective. The four questions are:

- What have we tried?
- What have we learned?
- What are we pleased about?
- What are we concerned about?

Plus one more:

- What does that mean we need to do differently?

When working with a woman who had Down's syndrome and was overweight, the following information was generated when using this approach:

- *What have we tried?* We had tried the community learning disability nurse working with her on healthy eating, the dietician reinforced some of this work and given Helen a more detailed diet to follow. We had also tried a healthy eating group at the day service she attended.
- *What have we learned?* We learned that Helen understood about healthy eating and portion control but did not seem to be losing weight. What we also learned was that Helen liked to have support for anything she was attempting and lots of positive feedback – we knew this from the work she was doing with the Partnership Board. We also realised that Helen was not happy with her life and did not see the point in being healthy when she had nothing of value to do during the week and on weekends.

- *What are we pleased about?* Helen was pleased she knew so much about healthy eating.
- *What were we concerned about?* Helen was concerned she was not losing weight and she was not happy and did not value her lifestyle.
- *What does that mean we needed to do differently?* Along with Helen we decided that it was more important to find something she would enjoy doing both during the week and at weekends and some friends to do this with. Having realised how important this was to Helen, it became very apparent that she would not be successful with her healthy eating and weight loss until this was resolved.

Over the next few months we managed, by using a direct payment, to change things for Helen. She now has a variety of things she likes to do during the week including attending the local People First group and spends some time with her friends from there on a weekend. Since sorting all this out Helen has been much more motivated to eat healthily and she has now started to lose weight.

Communication charts

These are described in detail in Chapter 7. In the context of a person's health they are useful, for example, when working with a person who has little communication but has frequent health needs. They can be particularly useful when describing what a person does if they are in pain (see Table 6.3), or about to have a seizure. Whether the person has a separate communication chart purely for their health-related issues is a moot point, it would, however, probably be more effective if they had one communication chart that included relevant health issues within it.

Table 6.3 Sean's health communication chart

What is happening/ where/when?	Sean does . . .	We think it means . . .	And we should . . .
This can happen at any time so careful observation of Sean is needed. Check he is alright whenever you are near him or in his company	Sean holds his hand to his head and his eyes look far away (see picture in his communication book) and he is hot	That he is in pain	Get Sean's communication book out and point to the different parts of his body to help him to tell us where it hurts. He will do this by nodding. Run a warm bath for Sean to help him relax and give him some pain relief. Sean needs this in liquid form.

Activity 6.4

What do you think the advantages and disadvantages would be of a separate health communication chart?

Having a separate communication chart for health issues would have the advantage of being able to develop it for a small defined group of people around the person and whose focus was health. In addition, it would mean the health issues were high priority for anyone seeing the chart. On the other hand, the difficulties or disadvantages could be significant. Having two communication charts could be confusing for people. It may mean that people operate with one and not with both. It would be time-consuming for the person whose chart it was to be involved in the development of both. It also means the health issues stay as an 'add on' rather than being central to the person's overall quality of life.

Learning logs
Learning logs can easily replace the majority of recording systems that exist within services. Most recording systems identify what happened, often in the context of antecedents, behaviour and consequences. While this can serve a purpose, the purpose is secondary to what can be learned via the use of learning logs. Learning logs are a useful approach to identifying what has been learnt in relation to any intervention or activity with the person. They can either be completed by the staff team, professionals working with the individual or the individual themselves (more detail can be found in Chapter 7). Whichever approach is used, the fundamental issue is about recording what was learnt rather than describing what happened. By recording what was learnt, lots of information that is important to and for the person is placed in the arena of those who support and care for the person rather than staying in the head of one individual who at some point is likely to move on from the focus person.

This approach has a number of advantages: it means that information can be built on cumulatively with the possible outcome of improving the person's life, and if we are doing this with a focus upon health, then ultimately their health may be improved. This approach not only shares information with a positive outcome but also allows for the development of a learning culture around an individual. Problems or issues experienced by the individual and/or those supporting them can be resolved through identifying learning and acting upon this. This can lead to a positive environment in which people are supported to grow and develop. Table 6.4 presents part of Jake's learning log in relation to his management of his diabetes.

Table 6.4 Jake's learning log

Date	Activity (what, where, how long?)	Who was there (support staff, friends, others)	What worked well about the activity? What should continue? What did you learn?	What did not work? What must be different/changed next time? What did you learn?
11 Oct.	Jake pricking the side of his finger using his finger pricker	Jake, his Mum and Katie, his support worker	Jake was good at loading the pen. What he was not good at was knowing exactly where to prick to get the best drop of blood with the least pain and to give enough for testing	Jake did get enough blood to test for his blood sugars. But to get this he had to put pressure on the area and this was painful because he had pricked his finger too far from the side of his nail. Next time show Jake the best place to position the pen before he pricks his finger – down the side of his finger, near the side of the nail (see attached picture)
12 Oct.	Jake pricking the side of his finger using his finger pricker	Jake and Katie	Jake was better at his finger prick today because I showed him where to do it. He got more blood with less effort and said it did not hurt as much	To continue to talk about what Jake needs to do and where to position the pen before he starts the process

Decision-making agreement

This particular tool within the person centred framework could and should become increasingly important as a consequence of the Mental Capacity Act (2005 effective October 2007). A decision-making agreement enables a person to articulate what important decisions they make in their life, in this instance in relation to their health. It allows them to state how they would like these decisions to be made, who should be involved in making the decisions and who has the final say in any of the decisions. The how and the who will usually change from decision to decision. Table 6.5 shows us Sally's decision-making agreement in relation to some of her health needs.

Table 6.5 Sally's decision-making agreement

Important decisions in Sally's life	How must I be involved?	Who makes the final decision?
Healthy eating	I must be involved in the shopping, in menu planning and in preparing and cooking my meals. I need Andrea to help me understand what is good for me and what is not. Andrea can remind me of the outcomes of eating bad food but that is all. She needs to do this in a friendly way not an 'I know what's good for you' way	Me
When to be admitted to hospital	I have bipolar disorder so every once in a while I need to be admitted into hospital. To make this decision I need my mum to sit down with me before I get to the point where I start not eating properly and talk through with me what is happening and help me make decisions about what happens next	Me and my mum

Accessible information/total communication

Accessible information is a slightly different aspect of person centredness and one where much more progress appears to have been made in relation to health action plans. In *Valuing People* and the health action planning work a clear message was given that the format for the plan needed to work for the person and that there was no single way to develop a health action plan for an individual. While we have focused on making health action plans accessible for people, and many places have consulted with people who have a learning disability about the format of a range of documents designed to improve communication, knowledge and understanding regarding their health needs, in the main, professionals have opted to develop a format for the plan. Everywhere has a different format but nevertheless most areas have one. This is often an attempt not to miss anything out and in order to ensure that both professionals and organisations meet their duty of care. While this is not wrong, it does lose the flexibility that had been created in *Valuing People* and could in some ways make the integration of some of the approaches and tools we have discussed so far a more complicated process.

Whichever approach you are operating, it is essential to utilise the resources and approaches that are available to help people who have a learning disability have greater control over their health. Typical approaches include the use of the basic standards relating to formatting of documents, using pictures such as those in the Change; Health Picture Bank (www.changepeople.co.uk/ default.aspx?page=10139), photos and symbols such as those included in 'worth a thousand words' (www.photosymbols.co.uk) as well as approaches such as multimedia profiling.

Accessible information is in essence just one part of the much bigger picture of total communication (see Chapter 7), it is therefore important to consider the range of other approaches that can help to make health interventions more person centred.

Activity 6.5

How can you use multimedia profiling with a person to develop their health action plan?

Multimedia profiling is an aspect of total communication that can be used to show how to meet the needs of different people we provide support to, Table 6.6 is part of a multimedia health action plan for Steven.

This profile focuses upon Steven's diabetes and how this is managed, normally it is part of a PowerPoint presentation but for the purposes of this chapter it has been extracted from the multimedia presentation. An additional part of his health action plan is a 2-minute video that shows how Steven must be transferred from his chair to the floor and from the floor back into his chair. This video, which we cannot show here, goes everywhere with Steven and he shows it to anyone new he meets who will have any involvement in moving him out of his chair. Showing people in this way helps people to understand what needs to happen better and faster and in a way that keeps Steven safer. It is also more accurate than explaining it to people using more traditional care planning approaches.

Introducing, contributing, safeguarding and integrating

In addition to all the strategies or approaches discussed above, Kilbane and Sanderson (2004) identified a model that outlined the different ways that professionals could be involved in person centred planning. These approaches can also be considered in relation to health action planning, and particularly to integrating both. They are: introducing, contributing, safeguarding and integrating. Each of these aspects of working with person centred planning are discussed in more detail in some of the other chapters, most notably Chapters 2, 10 and 11. In this section we will explore the relevance to health needs and health action planning.

Table 6.6 Steven's multimedia profile

Medical procedure	Steven's profile
Insulin regime	• I take three injections of novo rapid insulin a day at breakfast, lunch and teatime • I have two long-acting injections, one in the morning and one before bed • I am able to take my insulin independently • If I am out, I may ask you to carry my needle as it drops out of my pocket • I often need reminding about my insulin before I go to bed as I often forget this
Taking blood sugars	• I should test my blood sugar levels at least three times a week • I am not very good at remembering this • I need people to ask me how my sugar levels are and this prompts me into doing it
Tablets	• I take my tablets three times a day, breakfast, lunch and tea • I can do this on my own and do not need prompting
Managing my diabetes	• If my sugar levels drop, I may go hypo • When this happens, I become stroppy, this is not intentional, it is just what happens • If this happens I need support to manage this, I need glucose quickly • I carry Detox sweets, most of the time I will need a couple of these • I will then need to eat something sweet like chocolate • I will need to test my sugar levels to see if they are increasing • I may need some time to sit and recover • I do not always follow the diet I should and sometimes my sugar levels are high • When my sugar levels are high, my sides and my shins begin to itch • If I start scratching, ask me if my blood sugar levels are OK

Introducing

In introducing the health professional or any other person might find the person unaware of the role that person centred planning is able to play in managing changes within their life. In this situation the person may find themselves informing the individual with a learning disability and their family about what person centred thinking and planning are, possibly the different types of planning, some of the approaches that could be used to help identify what the individual wants and how they wish to live their life, as well as putting them in touch with the local person centred planning team.

In relation to health needs and how these are met within a person centred planning context, the health professional may indicate which person centred planning tools usefully include health issues in order to facilitate the natural integration of the two. The final decision as to which is used is, however, that of the person. In addition, the concept of introducing can be considered in relation to health action planning. Some people still do not know about health action planning and so it may be useful also to introduce this to individuals. In this context it may be important to explain to people the overlaps and the differences between person centred planning and health action planning and the ways this may inform the person's decisions about how they wish to progress. It may also in some circumstances be relevant to introduce the concept of a health action plan forming the start of a person centred planning process.

Contributing

Within this aspect of the model, the professional or other worker may be invited to contribute by being at the person centred planning meeting. They may also pick up certain areas to work with the person on, as a result of the meeting, whether they were attending or not. They may also be asked to contribute by providing information relating to a person's health needs, either for the meeting or in advance of the meeting. Whichever way this operates, it is important that the information is acquired in a person centred way and that it is provided in an accessible format for the individual. In this way the goals of improving a person's health will not be at risk of being lost in the bureaucracy of 'we do it this way here'.

If the tools we have discussed earlier form the basis of any professional intervention, then achieving this should not be difficult. It is, however, that subtle difference between placing the person at the centre of your professional intervention, or, working with the person to understand what all this means for them.

In addition, a health professional may be asked to check a person's plan with regard to the health aspects included within it. This may result in them identifying issues that have not been included or some questions or issues that need attention. For example, John had very complex health issues and his health action plan was shared with a community nurse. She had concerns that John's plan described that he had his prescribed tablets crushed. Her insight made the facilitator aware that the question that needed to be asked was whether crushing the tablets might alter their combination or effect. In addition, the medication in this case was such that it required regular monitoring via blood level testing. The health professional advised the facilitator who realised no monitoring of the medication had taken place for many years. The community nurse was also able to highlight the need for a continence re-assessment and the reason why.

Safeguarding

Safeguarding the quality of the work around person centred planning is important. Person centred planning facilitators are human beings subject to the foibles of the rest of the population, it is therefore incumbent on all of us to ensure the quality of the plans is of a high standard. Health professionals can help by reviewing the health-related information within a person centred plan, as such, they are a crucial resource to work with person centred planning facilitators. The same issues apply to health action plans when those are separate from person centred plans. Again, this is everyone's responsibility.

In addition, we are moving towards using person centred thinking tools to embed person centred practices in service delivery, consequently the issue of safeguarding multiplies in its complexity. Some of the structures for managing and analysing this include professional networks, team meetings/ supervisions, group and individual supervisions and the development of communities of practice and membership of groups such as the International Learning Community for Person Centred Practice. All these structures have a part to play, as well as personal professional responsibility, to remain up to date with contemporary practice.

Integrating

This operates at three levels: an individual's direct practice, within the team and organisation that you work in and within your profession. The different forums you as a professional either find yourself in or able to link into can be useful to integrating person centred practice and health. Some examples of this exist and are discussed in other chapters, for example, Chapters 2 and 3 where the example is given of a person centred planning co-ordinator attending community nursing meetings on a quarterly basis in order to identify themes and problems with plans as well as successes to inform the partnership board and other structures. This is so that person centred planning is implicit in the work of the organisation. From a health perspective, there are a number of ways in which this whole approach can be more integrated. These include professional networks being informed about person centred planning and person centred approaches, skills and tools, as well as promoting their use.

While person centred planning is the domain of people trained to operate in this way, person centred skills and tools, as outlined in Chapter 3 and earlier in this chapter, are much more the domain of all of us. This does not mean we do not need training and support to implement them, of course we do, however, this training needs to be supplemented by a range of structures such as professional networks, team meetings and supervision structures. It is through these areas that we are able to safeguard the quality of how the tools, etc. are being used as well as integrating them into the everyday use of colleagues.

In order to integrate person centred planning and person centred approaches, skills and tools within the organisation as a whole, it is also important to identify all the possible linkages that are needed to achieve this. This will be different for each organisation but a useful starting point could be to analyse the decision-making structure of your organisation in order to identify where you need to influence in order to make the whole approach to meeting people's health needs more person centred. Having done this, it may be helpful to utilise the approach of identifying who in those structures will be allies or champions and will make this happen with you. The next group to identify would be those people who will help it happen, those who will let it happen and then those people who will resist. This allows you to work out where to best invest your energies in integrating these approaches into the work of your organisation.

Conclusion

Health is a crucially important area for all of us. Being healthy is what allows us to live the lives we want and in the way we wish to. This is no different for people who have a learning disability, this is why health action plans are very important for some people. From the perspective of people who have a learning disability, however, the difference is the vast range of professionals involved, all of whom have a view about how that person should live their life, what they should and should not do. This is reinforced by the fact that each of us as a professional are taught to look at the needs of the person in a specific way. This is often described as holistic but is rarely so, as is indicated by the differences in our professional backgrounds. It is for these reasons that it is important that we as health professionals embrace the opportunities afforded to us by more closely integrating health action plans with person centred plans and utilising person centred tools to develop health action plans that are not within a person centred plan. The final step we can also take is to integrate this range of tools into our overall way of operating as a professional so as to ensure all the work we do is person centred.

References

Department of Health (2001) *Valuing People: A New Strategy for Learning Disability for the 21st Century*. London: Department of Health.

Kilbane, J. and Sanderson, H. (2004) 'What' and 'how': understanding professional involvement in person centred planning styles and approaches, *Learning Disability Practice*, 7(4): 16–20. Available at: www.helensandersonassociates.co.uk

Moss, S. and Turner, S. (1995) *The Health of People with Learning Disability.* Manchester: Hester Adrian Research Centre.

Smull, M.W. and Harrison, S.B. (1992) *Supporting People with Severe Retardations in the Community.* Alexandra, VA: National Association of State Mental Retardation Program Directors.

Useful resources

Helen Sanderson Associates
www.helensandersonassociates.co.uk

Support Planning Website
www.supportplanning.org

7 Communication

Louise Skelhorn and Kim Williams

Key issues

- Person centred thinking
- Person centred planning
- Total communication
- Listening and hearing
- Communication maps
- Communication dictionaries

Introduction

> No matter how one may try, one cannot, not communicate. Activity or inactivity, words or silence all have message value: they influence others and these others, in turn, cannot, not respond to these communications and are thus themselves communicating. It should be clearly understood that the mere absence of talking or of taking notice of each other is no exception to what has just been asserted.
>
> (Watzlawick et al. 1967: 49)

As Watzlawick et al. (1967) illustrate, any individual can communicate and professionals can hear that communication if they listen hard enough. This is true for people who have no intentional verbal communication, as well as individuals who experience difficulties understanding communication, expressing information and utilising communication within a typical conversational context. In this chapter we will explore the essential connection between total communication and person centred thinking and planning, the legislative context for total communication and explore the use of the person centred thinking tools, particularly 'communication charts' and communication dictionaries.

The relationship between total communication and person centred planning

Total communication is central to person centred thinking and planning approaches. Person centred planning provides a structured framework for listening to a person's likes, dislikes, hopes, aspirations and fears. Person centred thinking skills and their associated tools underpin this framework. Person centred planning involves working closely alongside people (Croft and Beresford 1993), in alliance with their friends, families and paid supporters, to consider what is *important to* and *important for* the individual now and in the future (see Chapter 4 for more details of this approach). Implicit within the underlying principles of person centred planning and thinking is the absolute commitment by professionals (Boud et al. 1985) to continually listen to and learn with the person. Total communication is fundamental to the success of this and in ultimately creating meaningful, positive change in a person's life. Striving to develop a culture of listening and learning is crucial in realising a shift in the balance of power between the individual and the professional (Ramcharan et al. 1997). It is within the context of embracing this total communication approach that person centred planning is emphasised as a set of promises, acknowledging that what is heard depends on what is being listened to. It is a promise to listen. To listen to what is being said, to what is meant by what is being said and to keep listening. It is a promise to act on what is heard, to always find something that can be done today or tomorrow and to keep acting on what is heard. Finally, it is a promise to be honest, particularly when professionals do not know how to help someone achieve what they are asking for, when what the person is saying is in conflict with staying healthy and safe or a good balance cannot be easily found between what is *important to* the person and what is *important for* the person. Addressing person centred planning without utilising total communication approaches can result in the person's plan being impoverished.

Wilson and Beresford (2000) state that without this cultural shift, professionals are merely paying lip service to the potential of what can be achieved. As you will see throughout this chapter, the principles of both total communication and person centred planning have significant synergy and both can work together to enhance the potential inherent within the other. Before exploring these synergies in more detail, however, we need to explore some of the fundamental principles inherent within communication.

Activity 7.1

Why do you think we communicate?

Your list may include some of the following:

- to ask for what you need;
- to express your likes and dislikes;
- to express your opinion;
- to make choices;
- to reject something/someone;
- to ask for information;
- to respond to others' questions and instructions;
- to form relationships with others;
- to be understood and to understand others;
- to share yourself socially with others, both on a personal and a community basis;
- to express your feelings;
- to organise yourself and make plans;
- to solve problems;
- to praise;
- to criticise or challenge.

As you can see, there are many reasons why people need and like to communicate. It is one of the most fundamental human activities, which underpin virtually every activity of people's daily lives. Despite the fact that most of us communicate spontaneously, unconsciously, and with ease, there are numerous people for whom this presents a daily difficulty. Regardless of the person's overwhelming desire to communicate, these difficulties can be of varying degrees and present in a number of different ways. Each one raises potential difficulties for professionals and person centred planners when trying to ascertain a person's views.

While successful communication with people who have communication impairments may look very different, it is an attainable reality. It is even supported by legislation (Box 7.1).

As already stated, this can be achieved through the principles of total communication. For the purposes of this chapter total communication will be defined as:

> *a communication philosophy – not a communication method and not at all a teaching method . . . Total Communication is an approach to create a successful and equal communication between human beings with different language perception and/or production . . . To use Total Communication amounts to a willingness to use all available means in order to understand and be understood.*

> (Hansen 1980: 22)

Box 7.1 The legislation supporting the move towards total communication

---

The Government White Paper *Valuing People* (Department of Health 2001) identifies four key principles that should be at the heart of all services for people with a learning disability. These are facilitating and promoting choice, independence, social inclusion and civil rights. Clearly, total communication and person centred thinking impact on all four of these.

The Disability Discrimination Act (Department of Health 1995) targets the specific discrimination people with a disability face in the areas of employment, buying/renting land or property and using services and amenities, such as shops, libraries, launderettes and leisure facilities. Under the Act, employers are responsible for making environments as user-friendly as possible for a person with a disability. This is not just about access but also includes the need to make communication person centred and information accessible for any person with a disability, which includes communication impairment.

The Department of Constitutional Affairs (2006) guidance to the Human Rights Act 1998, states Article 10 is freedom of expression. This supports using the means of communication most appropriate and natural for individuals in order to achieve this article.

If total communication and person centred approaches are to be combined in a successful fusion, to be utilised across professional settings, it is important to have an increased understanding about communication and the different complexities involved.

Components of communication

This section considers the component parts of expression and understanding and within this the importance of non-verbal communication.

Initially, it is most constructive to look at communication in terms of levels of symbolic representation, as illustrated in the Communication Model (Salford Speech and Language Therapy Department 2001) (see Figure 7.1). There are two sides of this model to explicitly represent communication as a two-way process. The two aspects of language illustrated are *understanding* and *expression*.

Understanding refers to listening to what is said, observing the situation, facial expression, gesture and working out what it means. Expression refers to getting your own message across. With any message, one person *expresses* it, and someone else has to *understand* it. People supported by professionals have

COMMUNICATION MODEL

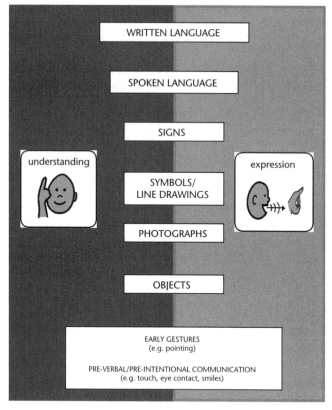

Figure 7.1 The communication model.

to take on both roles at different times and so do those involved in their support. The words in the middle of the model refer to different forms or modes of communication. These are presented in a general order of complexity, for example, it is easier for most people to understand photographs than picture symbols because they are more closely related to the real thing. Signs bear some relation to the real thing, for example, cup, whereas spoken words are a series of sounds and as such are completely abstract. However, as accomplished communicators, people use all these different forms all the time. Thus, it is implicit that total communication does not have a hierarchy of importance, preference or 'best', instead all forms of communication are equally valued. Total communication uses 'signs' to mean a formal system hand gestures and 'symbols' to mean pictures. Pre-verbal communication and early gestures are what enable us to have 'conversations' with young babies.

They are also important in adult communication. A great deal of information is gained from non-verbal communication such as facial expression, body language and tone of voice.

Non-verbal communication

In his studies, Mehrabian (1971) concluded that there are basically three elements in any face-to-face communication: words, tone of voice and body language. These three elements account differently for the meaning of the message:

- words account for 7 per cent;
- tone of voice accounts for 38 per cent;
- body language accounts for 55 per cent.

In straightforward communication, these three parts of the message support each other in meaning, that is they are congruent. In more complex communication, it is likely that incongruency, such as sarcasm, will be employed. The receiver of the message might be confused or irritated by two messages coming from two different channels, giving cues in two different directions. However, according to Mehrabian's findings it becomes more likely that the receiver/listener will accept the predominant form of communication (non-verbal), rather than the literal meaning of the words. So, in terms of sarcasm, it is the sarcastic tone of voice which changes the meaning.

Mehrabian dealt predominantly with communications of feelings and attitudes (such as likes and dislikes) and notes that the disproportionate influence of tone of voice and body language only becomes effective when the situation is ambiguous. Such ambiguity appears mostly when the words spoken are inconsistent with the tone of voice or body language of the speaker/sender.

Activity 7.2

Which members of our society may experience difficulties understanding incongruency?

These examples of incongruency are particularly pertinent to individuals who have difficulties understanding language, for example, people with the label learning disability, people who have had a stroke or are living with Parkinson's Disease or Alzheimer's, people who are spoken to in a language other than their first language and people on the autistic spectrum.

The Scottish Executive (2000) states that 80 per cent of people with a learning disability have a communication difficulty and 50 per cent have significant communication impairments. Therefore, non-verbal or pre-verbal communication can be very important in working alongside people with a learning disability and other marginalised groups. Individuals may be good at understanding pre-verbal communication, even if they are unable to understand spoken words. Consequently, it is possible to use supportive cues, such as facial expression, to help people understand what is being said. Individuals may also be good at using pre-verbal communication to express themselves. Indeed, Egan (1990) states it is essential that professionals be alert at recognising o9; and acting upon any non-verbal signals.

Activity 7.3

All communication involves comprehension and expression. This activity looks at what forms of communication Anna and John are using. For each scenario, decide if it is an example of expression or understanding and consider how that message is being conveyed. Reflect on what message is being communicated each time and by/to whom. Some have more than one message to consider.

1   Anna shouts 'Stop' to her son, before he runs in front of a bus!
2   Anna is waiting to cross the road. She sees that the lights show a 'green man' so she crosses.
3   Anna is on a bus and the man next to her lights up a cigarette. Anna points to the No Smoking sign.
4   John is at a party with his wife Anna. She taps her wrist and points to the door. They leave!

If you have considered each of the above examples you will have identified that the first situation is a demonstration of expression and spoken language, the second is understanding and the use of symbols, the third is expression, non-verbal communication and the use of symbols while the final example is understanding and the use of non-verbal language for John and expression and the use of non-verbal communication for Anna.

The skilled communicator

In order to understand and use language, certain prerequisite or foundation skills must be developed. In particular, skilled communicators must to be able to do the following:

- *Listen*: to noises, then voices, then words. Someone may understand the tone of voice, before they understand the actual words.
- *Look*: at faces and facial expression. This can be helped by signing, which draws people's attention to the face.
- *Pay attention*: to other people.
- *Take turns*: in actions, noises. This is how individuals eventually learn to take part in conversations.
- *Be interested*: in communicating and have a desire to interact with others.

Some people, however, may not have all or any of the prerequisite foundation skills that lead to skilled communicative competence and social interactions. As such, they may experience difficulties with communication. We will explore what this may mean for individuals and how to overcome some of the difficulties by looking at both understanding and expression.

Difficulties with understanding

People with a learning disability generally have difficulties with comprehension of language at some level. Individuals can vary enormously in terms of their understanding of language. Some people can experience great difficulty in understanding single words and may not yet have developed the foundation skills of communication. Other people will be able to follow complex conversations, but may have problems interpreting higher level language skills, such as sarcasm. It may be quite obvious when people have severe impairments with processing any spoken language, however, for those individuals who can process *some* language higher level difficulties can be hidden. The reasons behind this include:

- Supporters already modify their language appropriately.
- People use non-verbal cues such as gesture and routine to help them make sense of what is said.
- People may use learnt phrases, such as 'Hello, it's been lovely weather lately.' These can give the impression of better language skills than the person actually has.
- People become adept at using strategies to cover their difficulties with language or indeed behaviours, as it is often important to individuals not to overtly show them.

Some of these coping mechanisms are clearly identifiable in Rafi's story. He is a man in his late teens with a learning disability and profound deafness, who on finishing his secondary education went on to live in supported accommodation. His support staff, Jo, Pete and Naz, were concerned that he had an extremely restricted diet and seemed to be having coughing episodes at mealtimes. They had also noticed Rafi had lost weight.

Kim, a speech and language therapist discovered that although Rafi appeared to be chewing his food, in reality it was only his lips that were moving, not his jaw. Consequently food was building up in Rafi's mouth as he added more which eventually led to it falling into his throat causing coughing.

In restricting his diet, Rafi was trying to find foods that he could manage without explicitly asking for help and therefore revealing his difficulties. What became apparent was that Rafi had poor understanding and expressive language skills. Throughout school Rafi had adopted the persona of a 'helpful doer' so that he would not be required to understand or give information. His compromised efforts at mastering eating were therefore based on his observations of others. Rafi's downfall was that he only saw people's lips move and had no understanding of the motions and actions happening within the mouth.

Equipped with this knowledge and latest learning, Rafi and his support staff were able to develop an appropriate series of assistive techniques enabling Rafi to learn to chew, extend his diet and gain weight. Additionally information could now be relayed to Rafi at a level commensurate with his capabilities in understanding. Rafi's support staff also committed to using the person centred thinking tool, learning logs, (described in Chapter 6) to replace Rafi's usual notes (see Table 7.1). Learning logs directed Rafi's support staff to look for ongoing learning, within a structure that captures details of their learning around specific activities and experiences.

Rafi's staff used a learning log to record what was happening. Rafi and his staff concluded that through introducing assistive techniques alongside learning logs, they could track their efforts relating to this specific focused area for change and deepen their learning over time.

In addition to learning logs, there is a range of approaches that professionals can use to ensure they are supporting people in the best way possible. This section provides guidance on some of these and how to make yourself easier to understand. It also introduces the person centred thinking tool 'the communication chart' and 'communication dictionaries'.

The first step is to use total communication. Use any way possible to help someone understand. All the areas touched upon here will support people in understanding what is being said.

Say less
- Consider the person's level of understanding and the types of words and sentences appropriate for them.
- Simplify what is said – give the important information.
- Use short straightforward sentences.

Table 7.1 Rafi's learning log

Date	Activity (what, where, how long?)	Who was there? (support staff, friends, others)	What worked well about the activity? What should continue? What did you learn?	What did not work? What must be different/ changed next time? What did you learn?
20th June	Rafi was sitting at his dining table eating breakfast of Weetabix, banana and milk (20 minutes)	Rafi, Kim, Jo and Naz.	Rafi really enjoyed the Weetabix and mashed banana	Rafi did not enjoy the coldness of the milk. Next time warm the milk slightly to improve the consistency of the Weetabix and hence reduce coughing
11th July	Rafi was cleaning his teeth, with a supported programme of oral hygiene (2 minutes)	Rafi and Pete	Cleaning Rafi's teeth properly, including giving good attention to Rafi's gums and tongue. Pete supporting Rafi. Rafi's understanding of what is inside his mouth	Rafi found it difficult to manage the recommended 2 minutes of cleaning his teeth. Next time build up from 30 seconds and increase each time by 10 seconds, until the 2 minutes is reached

Stress
- Emphasise important words in sentences, for example, by pointing to appropriate pictures, objects or using signs.
- Repeat important words or pieces of information.

Go slow
- Some people find it easier to process information if it is presented to them at a slower rate. BUT . . . be natural, unnaturally slow speech can be more difficult to understand because the rhythm is lost.

Provide visual cues
- Show with real objects.
- Show with action, gestures, facial expressions and signing.
- Show with pictures.

Sentences
- Should be short.
- Should be uncomplicated.
- Should not include complex grammatical features.

- Should not include abstract non-literal language.
- Wherever possible, the subject matter should be within the person's experience. When this is not possible, use supportive material to aid understanding. For more details, see Box 7.2.

Box 7.2 Sentences

- *Long* sentences, such as 'Tomorrow I think I will go to the shops because I need some food for the birthday party that's happening at the weekend', will be hard to process. By the time the end of the sentence has been reached, the person may have forgotten how it started. Long sentences can usually be broken down into shorter ones, for example, 'Tomorrow, I am going shopping. I need some food. It is my birthday. I am having a party. The party is at the weekend'.

- How *complex* is the sentence? As well as the length of a sentence, reflect on *how many key ideas* are contained. For example, if someone is asked 'Can you go and get me a cup?' they may be able to respond appropriately just by picking up on the word cup. However, if the question were 'get the blue china cup for Sue', which is the same length, they would need to pick up on the words *blue* (not the red one), *china* (not the blue plastic one), *cup* (not the blue china plate), and *Sue* (getting it for someone else). This is therefore a more complex sentence. Speech and language therapists refer to this as the number of 'key words' or 'information carrying words' a person understands. Consequently, be mindful to reduce the number of key ideas in any given sentence we are using. Other aspects which make a sentence difficult to understand are *complex grammatical features* such as passives (the man was chased by the dog) and contracted negatives (there isn't any bread) which can easily be missed. Instead try using 'the dog is chasing the man' and 'there is no bread'.

- Is the sentence literal? In everyday conversation *abstract, non-literal language* is often used, for example, sarcasm. 'That was a clever thing to do!' And figures of speech, such as 'Pull your socks up.' These can often be taken literally, particularly by people on the autistic spectrum. This can lead to misunderstandings, frustration and potentially an increase in negative labels.

- *Subject matter*: Even when simple and straightforward language is used, it may be hard for someone to understand. This typically occurs when talking about anything outside of the person's experience, for example, situations, actions, events, behaviours, emotions. There is now an increasing range of supportive, educational literature, in a variety of accessible media. These could be used to facilitate discussions concerning particular issues outside the realm of an individual's experience.

Vocabulary
- Should be familiar.
- Have consistent word usage.
- Avoid abstract concepts where possible and support them with more concrete information when they have to be used.
- Should be motivating. For more details, see Box 7.3.

Box 7.3 Vocabulary

- How *familiar* is the word to the person? This will depend on the individual; some people will understand the word physiotherapist, because of their experiences. Others will not.
- Are words used *consistently*? For example, the same drink may be referred to by different people as squash, pop, juice, Ribena or blackcurrant. Some words have lots of different meanings. Such as, 'Give me a *hand*', 'My *hand*', '*Hand* me that cup'.
- Is it an *abstract* concept? Abstract concepts, such as time, can be very difficult for someone to understand, but words like tomorrow, yesterday, later are used frequently. Visual cues can be used to help people understand time, such as a diary or a timetable. Carers, supporters and family members also need to be consistent in their choice of words. Does *later* mean 'in 5 minutes', 'tomorrow' or 'maybe next week if not short-staffed'?
- How *motivating* is the word to an individual? People are likely to have a better understanding of words which are important to them, for example, chocolate or holiday. When starting to learn to sign introducing 'toilet' as a first sign, is not nearly as motivating as 'biscuit' and therefore less likely to be used or learned as quickly. This does not mean that the individual is ignoring the person using less motivating words; instead the person's preferences and interests should be considered as a sound starting point. Remember to always pay good attention to the learning environment. It is in knowing the person that best places their supporters, friends and family to phrase language in a motivating way for that individual.

An example of how important all this is provided by Jane, a woman in her mid-forties who has Down's syndrome. She lives in a supported tenancy with two other women and a team of 24-hour support staff. A speech and language therapy assessment of Jane's language skills was requested by her community nurse as part of an investigation into her behaviour. Jane's staff felt her behaviour was difficult to manage and wilfully obstructive. They felt the situation had become untenable when preparing to go on a shopping trip they had explicitly said to Jane, 'Don't shut the door.' Jane did indeed shut her front door, thus locking herself, her fellow housemates and the staff out!

On assessment it transpired that in actual fact Jane had no understanding of contracted negatives such as don't and had therefore correctly for her understanding, done exactly as she was asked and 'shut the door'.

Consequently the staff adopted the total communication approaches and the person centred thinking tool, communication charts. This was part of their ongoing learning and commitment to support Jane in a more person centred manner. Not least they stopped using contracted negatives with Jane.

Activity 7.4

What might have happened to Jane if a different professional specialising in any area other than communication had been called in to resolve this situation?

The profession is irrelevant in this situation, the important fact is that, had the involvement been from someone with a different approach, then the outcome may have been significantly different. The worst case scenario could have been one of Jane creating a career pathway for herself in which her life becomes a self-fulfilling prophecy and ultimately finds herself on significant doses of medication to manage her behaviour. While this may seem far-fetched, it is possible for it to happen.

Returning to the speech therapy involvement with Jane, one of the outcomes was her communication chart (Table 7.2). This provided an at-a-glance

Table 7.2   Jane's communication chart

What is happening/ where/when?	Jane does . . .	We think it means . . .	And we should . . .
Mealtimes, at home, with support staff	Jane is eating very quickly and spilling food on herself	Jane is hungry and had to eat quickly when she lived in the institution	Reassure Jane that she has plenty of time and no-one will take her food away from her. Gently prompt her verbally to eat more slowly. Do not say 'Don't eat so fast Jane', instead say 'Jane eat more slowly'.
Crossing the road to go shopping	Jane grabs at staff's hands	Jane is anxious about the traffic	Offer Jane an arm to link; reassure Jane that she is safe. Encourage Jane to use the pedestrian crossing and praise Jane for crossing safely, calmly and without grabbing. Remember to use positively phrased sentences. Avoid 'Don't cross now'; instead use 'Wait' and 'Cross now'.

view of key information about how Jane communicates and how to better support her during challenging times. Jane's staff felt that the charts were especially useful in supporting her as she communicates both through words and her behaviours. These approaches established a supportive system which ensured that Jane's communication is respected and valid.

Communication charts

The communication chart is a simple but powerful way to record how someone communicates with their behaviour. While this is a critical tool to have when people do not communicate with words, it is also important to use when communication with behaviour is clearer than the communication with words or when what people say and mean are different. Using the first person is more powerful, but it carries with it a responsibility. Only use the first person, when the person whose chart it is, is clearly in control of what is written in each column. In all other instances, the chart should be completed using the third person. Consequently, it is vital in developing any person centred plan where the voice of the person is being represented, that professionals begin gathering information with the people who know the person best and then check this out with others. The person's family are often the best people to begin with, or if they do not live with their family, then friends and the people who support them may be useful.

The first section of any communication chart, which identifies how supporters think the person communicates with others, has four headings:

- *What is happening*: this describes the circumstances.
- *What the person does*: in terms that are clear to a reader who has not seen the behaviour to the extent they would instantly recognise it. For people where it is hard to describe (e.g. a facial expression), a picture or even a video recording may be preferred.
- *We think it means*: describes the meaning that people think is present – a *'best guess'* is fine when the meaning is not clear. It is not uncommon for there to be more than one meaning for a single behaviour. Where this is the case, all of the meanings should be listed.
- *We should*: describes what those who provide support are to do in response to what the person is saying with their behaviour. The responses under this heading give a great deal of insight into how the person is perceived and supported. It is easiest to complete the communication worksheet by starting from the two left-hand columns first, starting with 'What is happening . . .', and then moving onto 'We think it means', and then working out to the two right-hand columns.

Another type of communication chart that can be developed (as illustrated in Table 7.3), is for use when people are using total communication to support a person who has different ways of communicating, including verbal communication and where people communicate through their behaviour. This approach can record how supporters involved in a person's life, are trying to communicate with the person. Instead of recording what the person does, the person's supporters can record what they are attempting to communicate to the person and furthermore, what they are encouraging the person to do. This type of communication chart has four headings:

- *At this time* this column is particularly useful when there are specific days of the week, or times of the day that need to be clearly identified and acted upon.
- *We want to let . . . know*
- *We do/say this . . .*
- *Helped/supported by . . .*

Table 7.3 Supporters' communication chart

At this time	We want to let Jane know . . .	We do/say this . . .	Helped/supported by . . .
	That Jane has made a mistake with her work/task/activity	Explain her mistake to her IN PRIVATE. Do not use contracted negatives, but show her how to fulfil her task using positive sentences. NEVER directly criticise Jane	Stay nearby in case Jane needs further assistance. Encourage Jane by telling her when she has done something well
	It is home time	Show Jane her 'home' symbol and reinforce this by saying 'It is home time'	Jane does not like waiting more than 5 minutes. After this time, support Jane by either reading with her or by sitting and talking with her. Jane also enjoys relaxing with her iPod on and needs assistance to start this running
	There has been a change to Jane's plans	Tell Jane as soon as you know, honestly explaining to Jane the reasons why. Use Jane's symbol timetable to show Jane when she will next be doing the activity/task	Be honest with Jane. Know that it is important to Jane to plan an alternative activity which she enjoys doing

Communication dictionaries and personal passports (Millar 2004) bring together communication charts and total communication. Communication dictionaries are, in essence, a synthesis of both types of communication charts illustrated in Tables 7.2 and 7.3. Communication dictionaries' value lies in the description of the minute detail of how a person communicates and their understanding. Like any person centred plan, a communication dictionary's strength lies in it being a living document which acts as a repository for past and present communication and future developments. As the person's communication changes, or indeed deteriorates, for example, as a result of dementia, the person's communication dictionary must be updated.

A personal passport, however, acts as a voice for a person to provide the kind of information we would usually find out when meeting someone for the first time. A personal passport is particularly useful to pass information from person to person; to act as an advocate for a person who has difficulty communicating; to ensure that people are consistent in their approach to a person they support; to help people during transitional stages, such as moving house, leaving school, going into hospital. Personal passports do not replace other forms of communication (speech, signs, symbol books). They are used alongside other approaches as part of total communication. For both of these total communication tools, the fundamental key is the process of gathering information.

Having looked at issues of understanding and what we as professionals can do to increase our ability to understand a person, it is important to now consider expression and the difficulties some people experience with this.

Difficulties with expression

People can have difficulties in expressing themselves through spoken language for a variety of reasons. If individuals have difficulty in understanding spoken language, they are likely to have difficulty in expressing themselves as well. However, some people with learning disabilities have developed effective social speech and learnt phrases, which reap benefits in terms of social contact. They can, however, hide difficulties in understanding.

- Many people with learning disabilities express themselves in *one or two word phrases*. This can be effective in many situations, but frustration can occur when the person wants to express something more complicated.
- It may be difficult for people to *find the words* they need. They may use general words like 'thingy' or words which are not quite right, like table instead of chair.
- *Articulation difficulties* can make speech unclear. Children and adults alike often find it very difficult to change the way they speak in

everyday life, so it can be more effective to look at other ways that a person can express themselves, to support their spoken language.

- *Fluency difficulties (stammering)*: This may depend on the situation, and the person's emotional state. Working on the fluency itself requires a great deal of self-monitoring and self-awareness, so it can be more effective to adopt strategies which support the person in their environment.
- *Use of language (conversational skills)*: People with apparently good expressive language skills may have difficulties in using their language appropriately, for example, people might make inappropriate comments or only talk about one subject repeatedly.

Activity 7.5

How can you support a person to express themself? What do you already do? What additional resources can you draw upon to significantly develop your skills further?

You can use a range of the following skills and approaches:

- *Use total communication*. Encourage people to use any way they can to communicate. Other forms of communication should be valued as much as speech. Ultimately it takes time and patience to enable people to express themselves, whether this is through speech or other means such as signs, symbols or objects of reference.
- People who stammer will be helped if they are given plenty of *time to speak*. It is not helpful to finish a person's sentence or to ask people to 'slow down' or 'think'. Instead lead by example, allow plenty of time, use a slower speech rate and try to create a calm, unhurried atmosphere.
- If the individual's message was understood, *accept how it has been delivered* – do not worry if it was not said 'correctly'.
- If someone struggles to find or remember a word, help them by *asking some supportive questions* such as, what letter does the word begin with or where would you find it? For example, in considering the word 'fork', the areas to ask questions on include things such as: What letter does it start with? Where is it found? What do you do with it? What is it made of? This is an obviously complex process and as such the amount of support and indeed the techniques employed are dependent on the individual. There may be a need to tailor this to be more or less specific, suggesting prompts to a greater or lesser degree.

It is also important to ensure that the person has opportunities to tell you that they have got it wrong!

- Have *visual supports* such as photographs and objects.
- Use *gestures and signs* as these can be effective.
- *Use strategies from person centred planning.* Learn from the person and from those who know them well. Ask questions that promote good conversations with people. To gather information, think about how to structure a conversation with that person and with other people who know them. While considering what will be learnt, be prepared to learn things that were unanticipated.
- In conversations:

    - Ask questions that are open-ended. For individuals who find free choice difficult to manage, then offer choice questions ('Would you like to live in a house or flat?').
    - Avoid questions that have a built-in answer ('Wouldn't you like to live with us?'). For people who are eager to please, their responses will incorporate what they think others want to hear (Smull et al. 2001).

Some good questions to ask an individual, bearing in mind that they may need to be tailored in accordance with the person's understanding and expressive abilities, are shown in Box 7.4

Box 7.4 Good questions to ask

- What makes a really good day for you?
- What makes a really bad day for you?
- If you had a magic wand and could have any wish come true, what would you wish for?
- What makes you laugh?
- What makes you angry?
- Who are the people you like to be with and why?
- What daily routines do you have? Are these different at evenings and weekends?
- How do you celebrate your birthday or special occasions?
- What would be your best holiday?
- What are your favourite possessions?
- What are the nice things that people say about you?
- What are you thanked for by other people? What compliments do people give you?

Talking Mats™

A total communication resource which enhances communication and helps people on their journey of decision-making, to think about issues and express their views, is Talking Mats™ (Murphy 1998). Talking Mats™ is a visual framework that enables people with a communication impairment to communicate more effectively, using picture symbols. Murphy and Cameron (2002) state that Talking Mats™ has potential for children and adults alike. The World Health Organisation (2001) describes a classification system which is a neutral list covering the full range of life areas, irrespective of a person's abilities. They are divided into nine 'domains' which can be used to support a person to examine an area of their life. Considering these domains ensures that all areas of life are potentially open to discussion. It is essential to think carefully about the options presented to any individual and a useful way to facilitate this is to use mind mapping (Buzan 1995). Talking Mats™ is a dynamic and flexible approach, as Figure 7.2 illustrates, which supports people to think about a variety of topics in different ways, including:

- getting to know someone;
- developing relationships;
- planning activities;

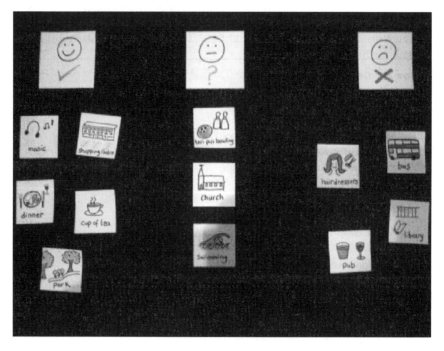

Figure 7.2   Planning daily activities

- to plan communication passports (Millar 2004);
- to enable involvement in person centred planning;
- to express views in meetings;
- to explore differences of opinions;
- to explore sensitive issues;
- to enable group discussion;
- to promote inclusion.

In order to not make limiting assumptions, professionals must reflect on what else they need to learn and know. In terms of inclusive best practice, professionals should be striving to integrate these approaches as every day tools.

Total communication and person centred planning as a way of meeting the cultural needs of people

It is imperative to be sensitive of and raise awareness of religious and cultural beliefs, which potentially give rise to differences in meaning (Ahmed 1994). A person centred plan must reflect a person's cultural belief system (Box 7.5). Any needs, routines or rituals that are associated with that culture or religion

---

Box 7.5 Meena's story

Meena is a young Muslim woman in her mid-twenties, who was planning to move into supported accommodation. Meena's planning facilitator Nazeem was mindful that Meena's religious beliefs were central to her daily life and as such her person centred plan needed to capture and celebrate Meena's interpretation of her faith. Meena chose Nazeem as her facilitator as it was important to Meena that her facilitator was a woman. Nazeem chose a person centred thinking tool to develop a greater understanding of what was important to and for Meena. This included an exploration of Meena's daily routines and rituals, both religious and personal.

In looking at Meena's morning routine the following richness of information emerged:

4.30 am *Meena wakes without switching the lights on for the Fahr prayer (early morning prayer, time varies throughout the year – usually 20 minutes before sunrise).*

4.40 am *Washes her hands. It is important to Meena to wash her hands followed by brushing her teeth and then to have a shower or ablution (wash for the prayer).*

4.45 am Meena first does the Sunnah prayer and then the Fahr prayer. Meena enjoys choosing the verses for the prayer, from a picture-prompted selection on a choice board.

4.55 am Meena sits on her prayer mat and meditates for a few minutes.

5.00 am Meena goes back to bed.

7.30 am Meena's support staff gently wake her. Meena has a lie in for about 5 minutes and then gets up.

7.35 am Meena goes to the bathroom and has a shower. Meena uses Dove soap, Pantene shampoo and Nicky Clarke's leave-in conditioner. Meena needs support with oral hygiene and uses Aquafresh mild and minty toothpaste and a small-headed Macleans manual toothbrush.

7.50 am Meena loves Vaseline body moisturiser and Body Shop vitamin E facial moisturiser as part of her morning moisturising routine.

8.05 am After dressing herself for the day, Meena has a glass of water or pure fruit juice, mostly orange, apple or cranberry (Meena does not drink tea or coffee). She enjoys two rounds of wholemeal bread, toasted, with Country Life unsalted butter for her breakfast.

8.30 am Meena says 'Salaam' to her support worker, picks up her handbag and day bag; puts on her hijab and headscarf and leaves for her work placement.

should be incorporated throughout the plan. However, be aware of making limiting assumptions with regard to an individual's cultural and ethnic diversity, experience or background (Wilson and Beresford 2000), if in doubt, ask the person or their family.

Total communication, person centred thinking skills and tools

When integrating person centred thinking skills and total communication, remember what is being explored is supporting people to have better lives, not just the development of great plans. The outcome here is not the plan, but the improved quality of life the person is living. In supporting self-determination, it is helpful to support people to think about and experience different opportunities. Professionals have a role in empowering people to proactively develop meaningful descriptions of how they want to live. Coleridge (1993) suggests that this must involve supporting positive change in terms of what individuals are doing and how they do it. This role must be extended to support people in their evolving vision of how and where they may wish to live and where relevant, with whom (Smale et al. 1993). Knowing what a person wants requires that any relevant people involved in support, learn and sort what is *important to* a person (what makes individuals happy, content, fulfilled) from what is *important for* (health and safety, being valued) the person, while working towards a balance between the two (Box 7.6). According to Smull and Sanderson (2005), this is a fundamental skill.

Determining paid supporters' roles and identifying specific responsibilities are always done by looking at what is important to and for someone, so that more than health and safety issues are taken into account. Using the 'doughnut' (as described in Chapter 3) can clarify the role of different professionals and agencies in supporting people. It also supports the development of professional creativity and lateral thinking; if people are to get better lives, supporters, planning facilitators and professionals must know where they can be creative without fear. Where there is a good match between the person being supported and the paid supporters, the frequency of labelled 'challenging behaviours' and the amount of staff turnover can be significantly reduced.

One of the most important person centred thinking skills is learning, using and recording how people communicate. Communication charts can provide a clear and concise overview of how someone communicates and can be especially helpful when supporting people who are pre-verbal and/or where

---

Box 7.6 Questions to consider when using person centred planning

It is particularly pertinent when beginning the development of a person centred plan to explore the following:

- Who knows the person well? Map out who is in the person's life to include friends, people from school/college/work; friends/neighbours, community members and religious or cultural leaders; people at home; family members.
- What makes a good day or a bad day?
- What are the person's routines and rituals? Remembering to acknowledge cultural diversity and clearly and concisely outlining specific details is key here.
- Do we know/how do we find out what a person's dreams and aspirations are?
- What are the person's needs and wants? Bear in mind that needs can often be very different from what a person may want.
- Does the person have what is important to them in everyday life, including people, activities, possessions and places?
- How do we support the person to stay safe and healthy (on their own terms)?

their behaviour communicates more clearly than their words. Where people do not use words to talk or where they communicate more clearly with their behaviour, recording their communication and using what is learned is critical (Smull et al. 2005). Communication charts can take a 'whole body' approach to communication. There are a number of other techniques which can be used for this, within a total communication approach. They include intensive interaction (Nind and Hewett 1994), individualised sensory environments (ISE) (Bunning 1998) and the Disability Distress Assessment Tool (DisDAT) (Regnard et al. 2007).

Conclusion

The integration of total communication and person centred thinking approaches means that professionals engaging with individuals *must* adopt an empowering, holistic, inclusive and person centred approach to any inter-action with the individual. Collectively, these are anti-oppressive in nature (Dalrymple and Burker 1995; Dominelli 1998). In addition, this means in prac-tice that an individual's communication, whether that includes any or all of the following: speech (*any* verbal language or vocalisations), sign language, symbols, pictures, objects of reference or the written word needs to be used and accepted within any aspect of their daily life. This includes an individual's environment, culture and their community, whatever that is to the individual.

Fundamentally, common sense is one of the most important tools anyone will need when it comes to thinking about communication. It is imperative within the context of using Person Centred Thinking skills, that professionals are able to both recognise and 'sort' what is *important to* someone and what is *important for* someone. The dilemma then is to creatively find the balance between the two, with the person and in alliance with the person's loved ones, family, friends and paid support (Smull and Sanderson 2005). What has been demonstrated here is that there can be no person centredness and/or planning without embracing the total communication approach.

Acknowledgements

The authors would like to thank friends and colleagues who have offered their support and contributions and all of the individuals who contributed to this chapter by way of providing the examples of the real-life events. Their names have been changed to safe-guard people's identity in accordance with their wishes. The authors would particularly like to acknowledge and thank Salford Primary Care Trust Speech and Language Therapy Department for sharing their resources and invaluable experience.

Symbols used in Figure 7.1 are courtesy of Mayer-Johnson Inc. Used with permission. Copyright © Mayer-Johnson www.mayer-johnson.com

Annotated bibliography

Nicola Grove and Barbara McIntosh (2005) *Communication for Person Centred Planning*. London: Foundation for Learning Disabilities.
This is an excellent resource in its own right and has an extensive resource listing, which would give the reader a well-rounded, broad base on which to further their knowledge and expand their insight.

MENCAP (2002) *Am I Making Myself Clear?* London: MENCAP.
This is MENCAP's excellent guidance for accessible writing. It is copyright free and freely downloadable from http://www.mencap.org.uk/download/making_myself_clear.pdf

Michael W. Smull and Helen Sanderson with Charlotte Sweeney, Louise Skelhorn, Amanda George, Mary Lou Bourne and Michael Steinbeck (2005) *Essential Lifestyle Planning for Everyone*. The Learning Community: Essential Lifestyle Planning.
This second edition facilitator's handbook pushes the boundaries of inclusive Essential Lifestyle Planning. This edition moves from a focus on plans for people with disabilities, to plans for everyone who wants one, including children and families, people with mental health issues, older people and people who have drug and alcohol issues.

References

Ahmed, S. (1994) Anti-racist social work: a black perspective, in C. Hanvey and T. Philpots (eds) *Practising Social Work*. London: Routledge.
Boud, K., Keogh, R. and Walker, D. (1985) *Reflection: Turning Experience into Learning*. London: Kogan Page.
Bunning, K. (1998) To engage or not to engage? Affecting the interactions of learning disabled adults. *International Journal of Language and Communication Disorders*, 33: 386–91.
Buzan, T. (1995) *The Mind Map Book*. London: BBC Books.
Coleridge, P. (1993) *Disability, Liberation and Development*. Oxford: Oxfam Publications.
Croft, S. and Beresford, P. (1993) *Citizen Involvement: A Practical Guide for Change*. London: Macmillan.
Dalrymple, J. and Burker, B. (1995) *Anti-Oppressive Practice: Social Care and the Law*. Buckingham: Open University Press.

Department of Constitutional Affairs (2006) *A Guide to the Human Rights Act 1998*, 3rd edn. London: Department for Constitutional Affairs: Justice, Rights and Democracy.

Department of Health (1995) *Disability Discrimination Act*. London: HMSO.

Department of Health (2001) *Valuing People: A New Strategy for Learning Disability for the 21st Century*. London: Department of Health.

Department of Health (2005) *Mental Capacity Act*. London: HMSO.

Dominelli, L. (1998) Anti-oppressive practice in context, in R. Adams, L. Dominelli and M. Payne (eds) *Social Work: Themes, Issues and Critical Debates*. Basingstoke: Macmillan.

Duffy, S. (2005) *Keys to Citizenship*, 2nd edn. Birkenhead: Paradigm.

Egan, G. (1990) *The Skilled Helper: A Systematic Approach to Effective Helping*. 4th edn. Belmont, CA: Wadsworth Inc.

Hansen, B. (1980) *Aspects of Deafness and Total Communication in Denmark*. Copenhagen: The Centre for Total Communication.

Kennedy, J., Sanderson, H. and Wilson, H. (2002) *Friendship and Community: Practical Strategies for Making Connections in Communities*. Manchester: North West Training and Development Team.

Mehrabian, A. (1971) *Silent Messages*. Belmont, CA: Wadsworth Inc. www.en.wikipedia.org/wiki/Albert_Mehrabian.htm accessed 7 Sept 2006.

Millar, S. (2004) *Personal Communication Passports*. CALL Centre Information Sheet 5, Edinburgh: Call Centre.

Murphy, J. (1998) *Talking Mats*. Stirling: University of Stirling, AAC Research Team.

Murphy, J. and Cameron, L. (2002) *Talking Mats and Learning Disability*. Stirling: University of Stirling, AAC Research Team.

Nind, M. and Hewett, D. (1994) *Access to Communication: Developing the Basics of Communication with People with Severe Learning Disabilities through Intensive Interaction*. London: David Fulton.

O'Brien, J. and Lovett, H. (1992) *Finding a Way towards Everyday Lives: The Contribution to Person Centred Planning*. Harrisburg, PA: Pennsylvania Office of Mental Retardation.

Ramcharan, P., Roberts, G., Grant, G. and Borland, J. (1997) Citizenship, empowerment and everyday life: ideal and illusion in the new millennium, in P. Ramcharan, G. Roberts, G. Grant and J. Borland (eds) *Empowerment in Everyday Life*. London: Jessica Kingsley.

Regnard, C., Reynolds, J., Watson, B., Matthews, D., Gibson, L. and Clarke, C. (2007) Understanding distress in people with severe communication difficulties: developing and assessing the Disability Distress Assessment Tool, *Journal of Intellectual Disability Research*, 51(4): 277–92.

Salford Speech and Language Therapy Department (2001) *Communication Model*. Salford.

Scottish Executive (2000) *The Same as You? A Review of Services for People with Learning Disabilities*. Edinburgh: Scottish Executive.

Smale, G., Tuson, G., Biehal, N. and Marsh, P. (1993) *Empowerment, Assessment, Care Management and the Skilled Worker*. London: HMSO.

Smull, M. and Sanderson, H. (2005) Person centred thinking, in M. Smull, H. Sanderson, with C. Sweeney, L. Skelhorn, A. George, M.L. Bourne and M. Steinbruck (eds) *Essential Lifestyle Planning for Everyone*. Manchester: The Learning Community.

Smull, M., Sanderson, H. with Allen, B. (2001) *Essential Lifestyle Planning: A Handbook for Facilitators*. Manchester: North West Training and Development Team.

Smull, M., Sanderson, H. with Sweeney, C., Skelhorn, L., George, A., Bourne, M.L. and Steinbruck, M. (2005) *Essential Lifestyle Planning for Everyone*. Manchester: The Learning Community.

Watzlawick, P., Beavin, J.H. and Jackson, D.D. (1967) *Pragmatics of Human Communication*. New York: W. W. Norton & Co.

Wilson, A. and Beresford, P. (2000) Anti-oppressive practice: emancipation or appropriation?. *British Journal of Social Work*, 30: 553–73.

World Health Organisation (2001) *International Classification of Functioning, Disability and Health*. Geneva: World Health Organisation.

8 Meeting the needs of people from diverse backgrounds through person centred planning

Chris Hatton, Nizakat Khan and Nji Oranu

Key issues

- The effectiveness of person centred planning for people from minority ethnic communities
- Evidence base supporting the use of person centred planning with people from minority ethnic communities
- Five dimensions of person centred planning
- Practical approaches to person centred planning with diverse groups of people and their families
- Strategic responses required to make person centred planning a reality for people who have a learning disability

Introduction

Like UK society as a whole, the UK population of people with learning disabilities is rapidly becoming more diverse. People with learning disabilities and their families who are from minority ethnic communities are often less likely to be aware of service supports, despite higher levels of disadvantage and a greater need for support, In addition, they are less likely to receive a wide range of services, particularly services that respect the language, religious and cultural needs of individuals.

In order to address this imbalance, this chapter tries to address three important questions:

1   Can person centred planning deliver where more traditional service support models have failed people from minority ethnic communities?

2   Do the values and processes underpinning person centred planning work equally well for everyone in UK society?
3   What practical steps will maximise the chances of successful person centred planning with diverse groups of people with learning disabilities and their families?

Diversity within the UK

The UK is becoming an increasingly diverse society.[1] For example, in 2001 8.3 per cent of people in the UK were born overseas, compared to 4.2 per cent of people in 1951 (National Statistics Online 2005). The number of people in Great Britain from minority ethnic communities increased by 53 per cent from 1991 to 2001, with 7.9 per cent of people in the UK (4.6 million people) from a minority ethnic group in 2001 (National Statistics Online 2003a). There is also diversity in terms of religion. In Great Britain in 2001 71.6 per cent of people identified themselves as Christian, 23.2 per cent of people either said they had no religion or did not state their religion, and 5.2 per cent of people reported belonging to a wide range of other religions (National Statistics Online 2003b). Unsurprisingly, the number of people with learning disabilities in the UK is also rising substantially (Emerson and Hatton 1999), with a projected increase of 70 per cent in the numbers of people with learning disabilities from minority ethnic communities from 1991 to 2021.

Activity 8.1

• How would you describe your ethnic origin and religion?
• What values would you say are important to you?
• Has there been a time in your life when your values have not been respected by others, how did you feel about this, and what did you do?

Although there are wide variations both within and between ethnic groups, it is beyond doubt that people from minority ethnic communities living in the UK generally experience substantial inequalities, discrimination and disadvantage. People from minority ethnic communities are more likely than their white peers to live in poor housing, be unemployed, be working in semi-skilled or unskilled jobs (if employed), experience poorer physical and mental health, and experience discrimination in education, health and social services (Modood et al. 1997; Nazroo 1997, 1998).

This experience of disadvantage is magnified for people with learning disabilities and their families who are from minority ethnic communities (Mir et al. 2001; Hatton 2002; Emerson et al. 2005; Mir and Raghavan 2005). They often experience disadvantage in terms of housing, employment, transport, income and benefits compared to white families with a person with learning disabilities (Chamba et al. 1999), who are themselves a disadvantaged group (Beresford 1995).

As people with learning disabilities and their families are often in disadvantaged circumstances with little support from extended family or friends, it is not surprising that parents report needing support from services (Chamba et al. 1999; Mir et al. 2001). However, they are much less likely to receive a whole range of services at all, let alone services that meet the needs of the person and their family (Mir et al. 2001; Hatton 2002). Commonly reported hurdles to accessing much needed support through service agencies include:

- service professionals not having the language skills needed to communicate with some people with learning disabilities and their families;
- information about service supports not being accessible to many people with learning disabilities and their families from minority ethnic communities, resulting in low awareness of potential support options;
- previous experience of services provided that either do not meet or actively violate the cultural and religious values of people and their families;
- racism and discrimination encountered within service settings;
- encountering an exclusively white workforce.

(Mir et al. 2001)

Similar issues have been reported for almost 20 years (Baxter et al. 1990). Despite recent policy initiatives to improve the way that services work with people with learning disabilities from minority ethnic communities (Department of Health 2001; Valuing People Support Team 2004), there are serious doubts about the extent to which these initiatives are having a real impact on people's lives (Greig 2005; Hatton 2005). This is of particular concern given the statutory duties incumbent upon public services in terms of race and disability equality (Shah and Hatton, in press).

In the UK, an increasing number of services are seeing person centred planning as a promising way of addressing the inequalities in access to appropriate support experienced by people with learning disabilities and their families from minority ethnic communities. Filomena's story (Box 8.1) demonstrates a positive outcome from such involvement (Hatton 2006).

Box 8.1 Filomena's story

Filomena is a young black woman of Afro-Caribbean decent; Filomena lived with her mother. Filomena's positive reputation was endless, those who know and care about her say that she is friendly, polite, caring and organised. Filomena has learning difficulties, she is employed in Asda, she is a committed employee, is never late to work and works really hard.

Filomena wanted to move into her own flat in the community, and had all the skills to do so. Her care manager from the 'Move on team' undertook the task of identifying a home for Filomena. Filomena was helped to make her Essential Lifestyle Plan; Filomena had two versions, one with lots of pictures and another with more words to it. Filomena and her facilitator who was an occupational therapist took lots of pictures.

Filomena's plan was ongoing but the search for a home was taking a long time, Filomena did not want to live with anyone. With the support of her facilitator they identified the kind of flat that Filomena would be happy to live in and what was important to and for Filomena. For example, health and safety issues were considered, Filomena was clear that she never stayed out late and was usually always home before 9 pm and on the odd occasion sometimes 10 pm.

All Filomena could focus on was her move . . . this became the main focus of her plan and subsequently more pressure was put on those responsible for making her dream a reality. Filomena's plan, with the help of her circle, focused on the support she would need to live independently, for example, she would need someone to help her to pay her bills. Filomena's plan also identified what she needed to learn in preparation for her move, for example, how to use the cooker and ignite the cooker, with her occupational therapist using coloured stickers to show which burner to light.

Filomena moved into a one-bedroom purpose-built flat in the heart of Hackney, with a concierge manned by a friendly security firm. Filomena's family helped her to decorate and furnish the flat. The flat is well situated for transport links and is easy for Filomena to get to work. Filomena was supported to learn her new bus route to work.

Filomena's story shows how a circle of support and person centred plan can focus people's efforts and bring about positive outcomes for people, particularly where things seem to be drifting.

What does the evidence base tell us?

The first question we have set ourselves in this chapter is: Can person centred planning deliver where more traditional service support models have failed people from minority ethnic communities? Unfortunately, the existing research evidence base does not help us to answer this question (for a review of the literature, see Emerson and Robertson, in press). Internationally, there have been few formal evaluations of the impact of person centred planning on people's lives, and those that have taken place have not investigated how well person centred planning works with people from minority ethnic communities.

The largest evaluation of the effectiveness of person centred planning to date has taken place in England (Robertson et al. 2005, 2006, 2007). Although this evaluation initially included 93 people with learning disabilities, only eight of these people were from minority ethnic communities, too few to investigate the specific experiences of people from minority ethnic communities. However, some of the findings of this study are important when considering the likely impact of person centred planning on people and their families from minority ethnic communities.

First, person centred planning had a positive impact on many aspects of the lives of people with learning disabilities, particularly in terms of improving social networks with family and friends, improving the number and range of community-based activities, increasing the amount of scheduled daytime activities and increasing choice (Robertson et al. 2005, 2006).

Second, 30 per cent of participants did not get as far as having a person centred plan developed at all during the lifetime of the study. The most common reasons cited for the failure of person centred planning to be implemented were related to facilitators, such as facilitators leaving or not being available. Professional facilitators themselves suggested that important factors hindering person centred planning included large caseloads and a consequent lack of time to spend planning with individuals, and bureaucratic procedures getting in the way of developing person centred plans (Emerson and Robertson, in press).

Third, there were variations in the benefits that different groups of people gained from person centred planning. For example, people with mental health, emotional or behavioural problems were less likely to have a plan and less likely to benefit from a developed plan. People with autism, people with more health problems and people with restricted mobility were less likely to receive a plan, but were sometimes more likely to benefit as a result of having a plan (Robertson et al., 2007).

Fourth, several factors were associated with developing successful person centred plans for participants. The single most important factor was having a facilitator who was committed to person centred planning; it was also important that people with learning disabilities took an active role in their own planning. For facilitators who were professionals, it was important that the facilitation role was recognised as part of their formal job role, that managers were actively involved in person centred planning, and that there was staff stability (Sanderson et al. 2006).

Taken together, these findings suggest that person centred planning should be a promising approach to working with people and their families from minority ethnic communities, although there may be additional barriers to its successful implementation. Person centred planning seems to be effective in improving people's lifestyles in areas that traditional services find difficult with people from minority ethnic communities (Mir et al. 2001; Hatton 2002). However, people with learning disabilities from some minority ethnic communities may be more likely to experience health problems and have restricted mobility (Chamba et al. 1999; Hatton et al. 2004a), factors that were associated with being less likely to have a developed plan. In addition, services may find it more difficult to find, train and support person centred planning facilitators with the skills, understanding and time required to engage in effective person centred planning with people and their families from minority ethnic communities.

Instead of waiting for an evidence base to appear, many services in the UK have proactively started to use person centred planning approaches with people with learning disabilities and their families from minority ethnic communities. Before discussing some of the practice-based evidence coming out of these service initiatives, it is important to consider our second question: Do the values and processes underpinning person centred planning work equally well for everyone in UK society?

Back to first principles

As well as considering the evidence base for the likely effectiveness of person centred planning with people from minority ethnic communities, it is important to take a step back and consider the values and processes that underpin person centred planning. If these values and processes are fundamentally incompatible in some sections of UK society, then the implementation of person centred planning could make things worse rather than better for these people and their families.

This potential incompatibility of values arises from a common view that person centred planning, with its North American roots, is highly individualist in character, whereas many sections of North American and UK societies may be considered as having more collectivist cultures (Emerson and Robertson, in press). Individualist (as opposed to collectivist) cultures have been defined by cross-cultural theorists in terms of:

1 The definition of the self as personal vs. collective, independent vs. interdependent.
2 Personal goals having priority over group goals.
3 Emphasis on exchange rather than on communal relationships.
4 The relative importance of personal attitudes vs. social norms in a person's behaviour.

(Triandis 1995)

So what are the fundamental values and processes that underpin person centred planning? Within the UK, the Department of Health describes person centred planning as 'a process for continual listening and learning, focusing on what is important to someone now and in the future, and acting upon this in alliance with their family and friends' (Department of Health 2002a). Five dimensions common to the wide variety of person centred planning approaches have been identified (Sanderson, 2000; Department of Health 2001, 2002a), and have been helpfully elaborated on by Brewster and Ramcharan (2005).

Table 8.1 presents these five dimensions of person centred planning, with a little more detail on some of their characteristics, and strongly suggests that person centred planning is capacious enough to be used in quite different ways ranging from highly individualist to highly collectivist and all points in between.

In fact, it could be argued that person centred planning is likely to be more suitable for people within collectivist cultures than traditional approaches to service delivery. For example, person centred planning's emphasis on the person is combined and seen as entirely consistent with a strong reliance on people's families, friends and community networks. Contrast this approach with traditional assessments of the individual's needs leading to the provision of services to supposedly meet these individual needs, with the individual's families and social networks being treated separately, if attended to at all. Person centred planning also reduces people's dependence on formal service supports (which are likely to be highly individualist in character) and opens the door to a wide range of informal community supports being used by the person.

In fact, Table 8.1 suggests that the major likelihood of cultural incompatibility lies not within the person centred planning approach itself but in the interaction between person centred planning facilitators and people with learning disabilities and their circles of support. As the description of person centred planning emphasises, facilitators need to bracket their

Table 8.1   The five dimensions of person centred planning

Dimension	Feature
Dimension 1: The person is at the centre of the process	The person is in control of the planning process. The planning group consists of the person and their circle of support (e.g. family members, advocates, friends, supporters). Membership of the group is chosen by the person, based on their relationships with other people. The ethos of the planning meeting is that the person is in control and has ownership of the meeting.
Dimension 2: Family members and friends as partners in planning	The ethos is of partnership with family, friends and people in the community, with professionals only invited when necessary. Conflict is resolved through the creative management of conflict through negotiation. The person and his/her circle knows best.
Dimension 3: Using the person's gifts, capacities and aspirations to judge the relevant support they need	The ethos is artful, creative and innovative in responding to wishes and dreams. There is a qualitative approach concentrating on total quality of life from the person's perspective. Information is presented in ways which are accessible and meaningful to the person and accessed by those involved in the planning.
Dimension 4: Planning for action	The focus is on a shared commitment to action in family, relationships and community as well as services to support these changes. There is a focus on mobilising resources in terms of those with a commitment to the person, i.e. communities of interest. There is a demand for a made-to-measure response from services and others.
Dimension 5: The planning process	Meetings: The plan is not the outcome. The circle of support meets as often as necessary. There is a continuous process of listening and responding to wishes as the person grows. Co-ordination: A continual process with the circle facilitator prompting relevant parties to act. Service orientation: Reflects what is possible. Still limited by service availability, but able to push for new services to cover an unmet need. A variety of formats running from the artistic and personal history right through to formal plans for action.

Source: Sanderson (2000); Brewster and Ramcharan (2005).

own assumptions and engage in a process of 'continual listening and learning' to build a person centred planning process that reflects the values of the person and those around them.

Activity 8.2

- Where would you place yourself on the individualist vs. collectivist dimension?
- What might happen if you took a highly individualist approach to developing a plan with a collectivist person?
- What might happen if you took a highly collectivist approach to developing a plan with an individualist person?

Wherever you place yourself, it is clearly important that you are aware of how this may affect your work with a person who has a learning disability and particularly someone from a minority ethnic community. This is especially important if you placed yourself within the individualist end of this continuum and you find yourself working within a culture that has a collectivist base to its beliefs and values.

What is happening in practice?

Although formal research evidence may be lacking, many agencies throughout the UK are using person centred planning with people with learning disabilities from diverse ethnic and cultural groups. These initiatives should help us answer the third question we set ourselves in this chapter:

> *What practical steps will maximise the chances of successful person centred planning with diverse groups of people with learning disabilities and their families?*

For example, an interim analysis of returns from a national survey of Learning Disability Partnership Boards in England (Hatton 2006) showed that 28 out of 72 Partnership Boards (39 per cent) reported person centred planning initiatives in their area that specifically included people from minority ethnic communities. The type of initiative varied according to the circumstances of different localities and included:

- For some localities with relatively small ethnic minority communities, using person centred planning on a small scale to offer culturally appropriate support, both with people currently known to services and to people newly in contact with services. This approach can help services to gradually build up their skills in offering person centred planning to diverse groups. In addition, it helps to gradually build community networks that both support person centred planning and identify new people not currently known to services.

- For a small number of localities with large and long-established minority ethnic communities, person centred planning initiatives for specific ethnic groups have been developed. These usually involve the employment of a development worker to establish strong links with the relevant community, facilitate person centred planning within the community and overcome broader barriers within service agencies to the successful use of person centred planning by people from minority ethnic communities.
- A more common approach taken by Partnership Boards has been to develop locality-wide person centred planning initiatives, but to ensure that the needs of people from minority ethnic communities are addressed within the general initiative. Ways in which Partnership Boards are doing this include:

  - ensuring that the people driving the person centred planning initiative in the locality are representative of some of the major communities in the area;
  - monitoring the uptake, use and success of person centred planning across ethnic groups;
  - ensuring that person centred planning processes have been piloted across ethnic groups and information is accessible to everyone in the locality;
  - ensuring that person centred planning facilitators (both professional and family members) include people from diverse ethnic communities;
  - working intensively within sub-areas that are particularly diverse in terms of ethnicity and culture;
  - ensuring that there is a robust link between person centred planning with individuals and strategic service development at a senior managerial level, so that lessons from individual plans can have a broader impact on services.

Activity 8.3

Considering the issues identified above, how many people from minority ethnic communities are using person centred planning in your area?

Are there more people from minority ethnic communities who could benefit from person centred planning? What can you do to make this happen?

The answer to these questions will vary significantly across the country with some areas having made more progress than others. Mohammed's story shows us just how important person centred planning can be in achieving culturally sensitive change for people from minority ethnic communities (see Box 8.2).

Box 8.2 Mohammed's story

Mohammed is a 27-year-old man who comes from a dual heritage background, his father is Bangladeshi and his mother is English. At present he 'lives' at a rehabilitation unit. Before this he lived at a nursing home for older people for eight years. His life there was described as very unhappy. People only attended to his personal care needs, completely overlooked his emotional and social life and also his spiritual needs were not recognised, respected or met in any way. Prior to his accident he was a 'good practising Muslim', a very helpful young man who assisted children to read the Quran at the Mosque. On a regular basis he would go to the Mosque and help in the cleaning chores. He was a popular member of his community, very caring towards his family and had a good relationship with his stepmother, brothers and sisters.

In the last few years of Mohammed living at the nursing home, his unhappiness became a growing concern to staff outside this establishment. He only ever had family visiting him, but he was never able to visit them. Although people who cared and were close to him understood and responded to his communication, staff totally denied his communication ability. Following an assessment undertaken by a social work student, many concerns were reinforced. One example was that he was being supported to go to Christmas carol singing, which was of no importance to him, yet no effort was made to assist him in celebrating his own religious festivals.

Assessment staff made a referral to the learning disability service to investigate his situation and find a way forward. A social worker and a link team co-ordinator (whose role is to ensure access is easy and barriers are removed for people from minority ethnic communities) began to work with Mohammed. Following their assessment and involving his family, they started to make plans for Mohammed to move out of the nursing home into supported living or a place where all his needs would be met. This was a challenging task, and following hard negotiations it was agreed that Mohammed's nursing needs were not being met anyway, which was the reason why he was at the nursing home. At this point an alternative was found.

At this stage, planning began with Mohammed and his family to ensure that a new basis for support existed that could be tailored around what was important to him and his family. Now Mohammed has a new wheelchair so he can go into his community and participate in things he enjoys. His family visit him twice a week and plans are under way to help Mohammed visit his family. People are getting to know his likes and dislikes so arrangements are made to assist Mohammed in doing the things that he likes to do. For example, he loves watching football and he is a keen Liverpool supporter. Planning meetings take place at Mohammed's on a regular basis, which provide more opportunity for Mohammed and his family to meet. Through planning his family are exploring possibilities for arranging a local Imam from the mosque to have contact with Mohammed. His family have brought him traditional clothes to wear on Fridays because this is an important day in the Muslim calendar. Mohammed's dream is to move back to Oldham and live close to his family, in his own home with support. His support circle is making efforts to find his close friends so that they can start to meet up with him again.

Staff who support him recognise his way of communication, and have increased their awareness and understanding. For example, arrangements were made to have an Eid party – this was the first time a religious festival meaningful to Mohammed had been recognised by the establishment. This highly successful event also gave an opportunity for making contacts with the Muslim community in the area, who have offered their support for Mohammed and other people who are in similar situations.

Currently the focus is on building a transitional plan to prepare for a move to his home town. From when planning first started, commitment and passion have grown through seeing the achievements and successes, inspiring people to believe that through working together it is possible to achieve the lives people desire for themselves.

Mohammed's family say: 'Planning has given us hope and a vision for a better future for Mohammed. We feel now we can have a say in how and what support he receives. We no longer believe that only professionals know what is best for our son. Mohammed's faith and cultural needs are recognised and responded to. We look forward to a day when Mohammed will move closer to us in Oldham.'

With Mohammed and his family, time was a crucial part of successful planning, with time needed to help to build relationships, trust and confidence with Mohammed's family as they had previously had very negative experiences of service support. Planning has also changed the family's view of their role, from one where professionals were assumed to know best for their son to one where they feel they have an important voice and role in their son's future.

Source: Abridged from Khan et al. (2004).

Person centred planning with people from minority ethnic communities

People who have used person centred planning with people from minority ethnic communities are increasingly sharing the learning from their practical experiences (Khan et al. 2004; Parmar et al. 2004). This final section of the chapter will outline some of these lessons, in terms of the issues involved in doing person centred planning with people and their families from minority ethnic communities, and the broader organisational and strategic issues that arise. Although this section will draw heavily on the experiences of Leicester (Parmar et al. 2004) and Oldham (Khan et al. 2004) when working with Asian communities, the issues and recommendations will be readily applicable to people from other minority ethnic communities and indeed will be of general relevance to anyone conducting person centred planning. For example, person centred planning around religious needs is likely to be important for a large section of the majority ethnic population in the UK as well as for many people in minority ethnic communities (Hatton et al. 2004b).

What styles of person centred planning might be useful?

People who have tried person centred planning with several people from minority ethnic communities suggest that the whole range of person centred planning tools should be available to person centred planning facilitators, as different tools and approaches are likely to be useful for different people in different circumstances (Khan et al. 2004; Parmar et al. 2004); more details on all these approaches are available in Department of Health (2002b), see also Chapter 4).

For some people who are in a position to state clearly what they want from their life, PATH and MAPs and personal futures planning may be immediately useful. These processes can focus thinking, ensuring that all key issues are covered and draw people together to solve problems. PATH and MAPs tools can help restore dreams and aspirations, and turn dreams and aspirations into specific goals as well as enrolling people in making the plan happen for the person. These tools might be seen as more spiritual and personal than assessment techniques and therefore difficult to bureaucratise.

Open planning is encouraged – to think literally and creatively in identifying sources of support. The tools must be used with skill, and heart, being able to truly listen to people's dreams and nightmares. Their hopes and visions must be captured in meaningful images. These are accessible to all people regardless of language, as they do not rely on words alone, enabling a shift of power to the person and the people who care about them. Assessments often do not touch on people's spiritual needs and wishes, but this tool enables a person to take control.

Essential Lifestyle Planning (ELP) is a guided process to learn how someone wants to live their life and help develop a plan to make it happen. An ELP is useful for anyone where it is helpful to find out what is important to an individual in their everyday life and to look at the support they would need and any issues of health and safety from the individual's perspective. ELP can be used in combination with other person centred planning tools. This way of planning separates what is *important to* someone from what others see as *important for* them. Developing a good plan requires us to reflect how people want to live, to reflect the perspectives of people who truly care about the person, to listen to what they like and admire about the person. All person centred planning tools require us to spend time with and listen to individuals and others who care about them.

Introducing person centred planning

Before being able to start person centred planning with people from minority ethnic communities, it is vital to prepare the ground so that people from minority ethnic communities can make informed choices about person centred planning. It is also important that facilitators with the relevant skills are ready to work with people from minority ethnic communities. Raising awareness is particularly important as many people may be generally unaware that service support is available, and may also be suspicious of another new 'service' that is being offered when previous services have been less than ideal.

In Leicester, an extensive programme of awareness raising for people and families from Asian communities was conducted (Parmar et al. 2004), including:

- the appointment of a development worker with the relevant cultural knowledge, language skills and knowledge of person centred planning to start talking to Asian people and their families about person centred planning – people and families identified this as crucial;
- organising regular events for Asian people with learning disabilities and family carers in accessible venues to discuss person centred planning;
- discussing person centred planning with community groups and community leaders in the Asian community;
- discussing person centred planning in meetings with independent and voluntary sector organisations that provide residential services aimed at Asian people with learning disabilities;
- investigating the provision of written information about person centred planning in a wide range of different community languages.

Leicester have also developed a rolling programme of training opportunities for person centred planning, ranging from introductory awareness raising, through to how to be a person centred planning facilitator and how to 'train the trainers' (Parmar et al. 2004). This training has been delivered by a mix of people with learning disabilities, carers and professionals to similarly mixed groups of people, with interpreters to ensure that the training is accessible to people using a wide range of community languages.

Activity 8.4

- What do you think would constitute good practice when working with people from minority ethnic communities?
- Are there things you can do individually to make your practice better?
- Are there things that require joint action to improve practice, and what part can you play in making this action happen?

Both Leicester City (Parmar et al. 2004) and Hackney (Oranu, unpublished) have produced very helpful checklists to consider when introducing person centred planning to people with learning disabilities from minority ethnic communities (see Box 8.3).

Box 8.3 Checklist for introducing person centred planning to people from minority ethnic communities and working with people in a person centred way

Names – are you pronouncing these properly?

Language – use of interpreters who are aware of person centred planning.

Find out about appropriate diet and food.

Find out about appropriate dress.

Washing and cleanliness – are these carried out according to the person's wishes, for example, the rinsing of dishes or personal hygiene?

Gender issues – for example, is there a preference for same gender support for personal care?

Find out about the person's religious beliefs and interests.

Find out about festivals that the person wants to celebrate.

Be non-judgemental – whose values are important in the person centred planning process?

Engage in active listening.

Consider the appropriateness of discussing issues of sexuality.

Show respect for the person's way of life.

Have some awareness of cultural issues that are likely to be relevant to the person.

But avoid stereotyping – recognise that individuals are not homogeneous.

Be aware of power differentials between the person and professionals.

Be aware of the broader context within which people live, in terms of discrimination and racism.

Show a professional commitment to antiracist, antidiscriminatory and anti-oppressive practices.

Khan et al. (2004), based on their experiences in Oldham, also offer valuable advice about what needs to happen for person centred planning to be successful with people from minority ethnic communities:

- When planning with people, it is important to make sure people/ families have good advance information around person centred planning so that they can decide if it is right for them and which is the right method or planning tool for their circumstances.
- Two trained facilitators are needed to do the planning because of language. One must be bilingual in the language spoken by the person and family.
- The facilitator has to have a good understanding and awareness of religious and cultural issues so they are able to ask appropriate prompt questions.
- A facilitator should not use an interpreter who is not trained or aware of the person centred planning process.
- Make sure that the graphic recorder is able to capture a true image of what the person is saying, through appropriate symbols.
- Families must be involved in the process, because they are often afraid that their issues will not be considered. In order to do this it is vital to plan with the person and the family and negotiate a balance.
- Time is an important part of successful planning; this will help to build relationships, trust and confidence with families to bring to life an effective plan with the person. Time is really worth investing – this results in a better understanding of the person's lifestyle and culture. This will better inform families of how to influence service developments and be more involved.
- While in the initial stages of planning, look at what is important to the person and the family. Take appropriate steps to link these themes into service development to bring about cultural change in the service. People can then see their plans coming to life and they do need to see early wins.

Taking a strategic view

As well as improving the lives of individuals from minority ethnic communities, implementing person centred planning can act as a stimulus to wider strategic changes across a whole service. Workers in Oldham have described how they tried to link the individual lessons from person centred planning with people from Asian communities to strategic change across the service as a whole (Khan et al. 2004) (see Figure 8.1). Figure 8.1 outlines the process by which person centred planning and other direct work supporting people and their families from South Asian communities in Oldham was linked to strategic thinking about service development.

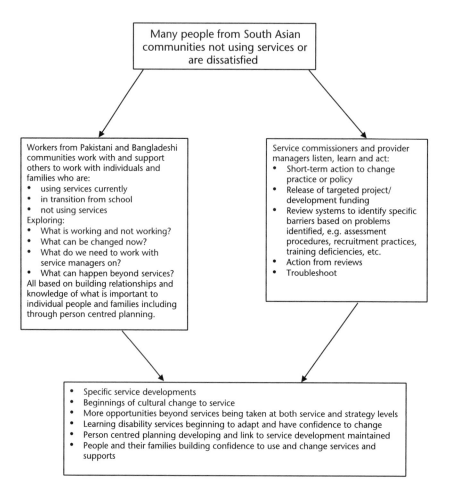

Figure 8.1 The Oldham model linking individual person centred planning to strategic change

First, careful and extensive research and outreach work clearly established that many people with learning disabilities and their families from South Asian communities in Oldham were either not using services or were dissatisfied with the services they were getting (the start point of Figure 8.1).

Second, an EMAP (ethnic minority action planning) group was established to plan and take short-, medium- and long-term action. This had good representation from across services and agencies and, crucially, senior management championing. Through the work of this group, and via senior management champions, close links were made to both person centred planning activity and to strategic service development planning (the right-hand side of Figure 8.1).

Third, a link team was established to act as a link between adults with learning disabilities, their families and services (the left-hand side of Figure 8.1). The team assists in the understanding of people's perceptions of services, and ensures that needs assessments reflect the norms and values of different communities and plans are developed and implemented accordingly. It links cultural factors and implications for service design and delivery with service strategy for change and development. The link team is a shift from an ethnically specialist support service within a service to a holistic/mainstream support, which promotes inclusive and equitable services for all.

Working together, some changes have begun to be seen across the service as a whole (the bottom of Figure 8.1), such as meaningful cultural awareness training for staff and the routine provision of same gender support for personal care.

Finally, Khan et al. (2004) offer some advice for professionals about how people with learning disabilities and their families from ethnic minority communities need to be supported so that they can effectively influence the services and supports they use:

- Good information should be provided about services in languages people understand, and networking opportunities should be made available to individuals and families to empower them in the process of their planning for the future (see Box 8.4).

Box 8.4 Hamad's story

Hamad is a 22-year-old young man who lives with his parents, two sisters and brother. He uses a day service a few days a week.

He went to a local special school. In 1997, the care co-ordinator began the transition process through spending time with him at school and at home with his family. Here came the opportunity for him and his family to look at what was important to him and what he needed to move into adult life.

Within weeks of getting to know Hamad, gathering information became very useful for his essential lifestyle plan. This helped us to plan as smooth a transition as possible. Hamad did not speak in words, and through planning together with his family and others who knew him well we developed a communication dictionary. This enabled two things, to understand how he communicated and to respond to his communication. We discovered that staff had very little understanding of how Hamad communicated, so therefore they could not respond to him. We made videos of Hamad in different situations to assess his likes and dislikes. This brought to our attention the fact that Hamad's wheelchair was extremely uncomfortable and unsuitable for his posture and needs. We found that he did not dislike all his activities; sometimes the reason why he would show dislike would be through his discomfort, caused by his wheelchair. When Hamad was asking for help in his mother tongue, staff would take this literally and repeat the sounds back to him, thinking they were encouraging a dialogue with Hamad. However, due to staff's lack of understanding of Hamad's likes and dislikes, and also not understanding his language, this led to Hamad getting frustrated to an extent where he became withdrawn and very upset.

Hamad's family began to become very keen on the planning process because some changes were made quite quickly. The plan resolved some immediate issues of support for Hamad at school, through getting a new moulded wheelchair and developing a communication dictionary, which when in place provided guidelines for staff who worked with Hamad.

At this stage the planning started to focus on transition into adult services. After tasters and introductions for Hamad and his family had taken place, they decided to start accessing a day service for a few days a week. Through working closely with Hamad and his family it was identified as an essential need for Hamad to have a same gender support worker to assist him with his overall personal care needs. This became an issue for debate due to the service not understanding that we could not and would not negotiate about the essential needs of a person. This would be a compromise on Hamad's faith and for his family. To them this was very important and was non-negotiable.

Through planning it also came to the forefront that Hamad enjoyed eating curries and spicy foods and was not particularly keen on plain food. At the day centre his dietary needs were in question because he was refusing to eat the food offered to him. This was for two reasons, one it had to be halal and the other because it just was not spicy.

The list of unresolved issues was beginning to grow rapidly. The care co-ordinator and others involved in Hamad's plan felt that changes needed to be made and also to look at everyobody's commitment to ensure that the plan happened.

Awareness training took place for the day service to look at cultural awareness and an insight into planning with people and what it involves. This was a necessary step because Hamad was the first person from a different background to access this service and also he was the first person to have an essential lifestyle plan. After the awareness training the day service appointed a worker from the same background and who spoke the same language as Hamad. When we offered resources to the service to guarantee Hamad's plan, it turned out that resources were not an issue, the issue was to be open to flexibility, to be more creative and to use existing resources in a flexible way.

Hamad's plan informed the service development strategy. Diet, personal care and gender-specific support were guaranteed for the first time in the service, and a link team was set up as a direct result of families wanting language support to come from knowledgeable workers.

Hamad's mum said, 'Planning has changed our lives, my son receives a service that guarantees meeting his personal and spiritual needs in the way which is important to him. We now have hopes and aspirations for his future. One in particular, which is to help him to buy his own house. Through planning it has equipped me as a parent to influence service design and delivery.'

For planning to work with Hamad and his family, it was crucial that his family was involved right from the start, as families can be scared that their issues will not be considered. As with Mohammed (see Box 8.2), taking the time to build strong relationships with Hamad and his family was crucial. Finally, lessons from some of the specific issues that arose with Hamad, such as diet, personal care and gender-specific support, were learned and applied across the service, benefiting many other people as well as Hamad individually.

Source: Abridged from Khan et al. (2004).

- Training should be made available in a range of relevant languages, and support offered through training so that individuals and families can lead their own planning.
- Support should be available for individuals and families through planning meetings from staff who understand their cultural background and bilingual workers who are trained in person centred planning.
- Staff should assist families in gaining information about non-specialist services, bringing about more choices and opportunities. This would also encourage partnership working with local community members.
- Training in Person Centred Planning should be provided for individuals and families so they can decide which is the right method or tool of planning they would like to use.
- Independent and individual advice and support must be available. This could include facilitation of plans, advocacy and self-advocacy and other support, for example, bringing carers together, also making links with other carers support initiatives.
- Professionals from statutory agencies including care managers, care co-ordinators should work to ensure that their assessment practice is complementary to person centred planning. This can be done in a formal or informal way.

Conclusion

At the start of this chapter we set ourselves three questions that we were going to try to address:

1   Can person centred planning deliver where more traditional service support models have failed people from minority ethnic communities?
2   Do the values and processes underpinning person centred planning work equally well for everyone in UK society?
3   What practical steps will maximise the chances of successful person centred planning with diverse groups of people with learning disabilities and their families?

Although formal research evidence to help us address these questions is absent, the practice-based evidence of people doing person centred planning with people with learning disabilities suggests the following answers:

1   Yes, it can deliver where more traditional service support models have failed *if you get it right*.
2   Yes, the underpinning values and processes do work equally well for everyone in the UK, again, *if you get it right*.
3   The practical steps include having a range of people from different communities trained to deliver person centred planning, flexibility in the responses to people's needs, an understanding of different cultures and a strategy and resources identified to support the process of introducing person centred planning into a community among many others. Importantly – you need to *get these right* as well.

The cornerstones of person centred planning, *'[the] process for continual listening and learning, focusing on what is important to someone now and in the future, and acting upon this in alliance with their family and friends'* (Department of Health 2002a), are as important if not more important for people from minority ethnic communities, who are likely to have received a raw deal from services in the past, including stereotyping, discrimination and disadvantage from the very agencies that were supposed to be supporting them. Person centred planning offers a positive way forward for people with learning disabilities from minority ethnic communities, and there is enough experience from people who have done it to provide practical and inspiring solutions for people who want to try it for the first time.

Note

1   There are many aspects of diversity within UK society, such as ethnicity, culture, religion, language and sexuality. Largely on the basis of the available material, this chapter is concerned with diversity largely in terms of ethnicity,

culture and religion. Readers interested in similarities and differences in definitions of 'race', ethnicity and culture are referred to Hatton (2002) and Shah (2005).

Annotated bibliography

Khan, N., Rahim, N. and Routledge, M. (2004) Person centred planning and people from South Asian communities: some experiences from one locality. Available at Valuing People Support Team website: http://valuingpeople.gov.uk/dynamic/valuingpeople88.jsp
A detailed and inspiring account of Oldham's attempts to put person centred planning at the heart of individual and strategic change for people and their families from South Asian communities.

Parmar, R., Brown, J., Shelton, C. and Potter, M. (2004) *Person Centred Planning with People from Leicester's Asian Communities*. Leicester: Leicester City Social Care and Health Department. Available at: http://valuingpeople.gov.uk/dynamic/valuingpeople88.jsp
A detailed account of Leicester City's initiatives to use person centred planning with Asian people with Leicester, but also filled with lots of good practice advice and guidance.

Robertson, J., Emerson, E., Hatton, C., Elliott, J., McIntosh, B., Swift, P., Krijnen-Kemp, E., Towers, C., Romeo, R., Knapp, M., Sanderson, H., Routledge, M., Oakes, P. and Joyce, T. (2005) *The Impact of Person Centred Planning: A Report to the Department of Health*. Lancaster: Institute for Health Research, Lancaster University. Available at: www.lancs.ac.uk/fass/ihr/research/learning/projects/person.htm
A comprehensive report of the biggest evaluation to date of person centred planning – although it does not say anything about people from minority ethnic communities!

Valuing People Support Team (2004) *Learning Difficulties and Ethnicity: A Framework for Action*. London: Department of Health. Available at: www.valuingpeople.gov.uk/EthnicityFramework.htm
A very useful framework for Partnership Boards to act to improve supports for people from minority ethnic communities – includes some information on person centred planning.

References

Baxter, C., Poonia, K., Ward, L. and Nadirshaw, Z. (1990) *Double Discrimination: Issues and Services for People with Learning Difficulties from Black and Minority Ethnic Communities.* London: King's Fund Centre.

Beresford, B. (1995) *Expert Opinions: A National Survey of Parents Caring for a Severely Disabled Child.* Bristol: The Policy Press.

Brewster, J. and Ramcharan, P. (2005) Enabling and supporting person-centred approaches, in G. Grant, P. Goward, M. Richardson and P. Ramcharan (eds) *Learning Disability: A Life Cycle Approach to Valuing People.* Maidenhead: Open University Press, pp. 491–514.

Chamba, R., Ahmad, W., Hirst, M., Lawton, D. and Beresford, B. (1999) *On The Edge: Minority Ethnic Families Caring for a Severely Disabled Child.* Bristol: The Policy Press.

Department of Health (2001) *Valuing People: A New Strategy for Learning Disability for the 21st Century.* London: Department of Health. Available at: http://www.valuingpeople.gov.uk/documents/ValuingPeople.pdf

Department of Health (2002a) *Planning with People: Towards Person Centred Approaches. Guidance for Partnership Boards.* London: Department of Health. Available at: http://valuingpeople.gov.uk/dynamic/valuingpeople136.jsp

Department of Health (2002b) *Planning with People: Towards Person Centred Approaches. Resource Guide.* London: Department of Health. Available at: http://valuingpeople.gov.uk/dynamic/valuingpeople136.jsp

Emerson, E. and Hatton, C. (1999) Future trends in the ethnic composition of British society and among British citizens with learning disabilities. *Tizard Learning Disability Review,* 4: 28–32.

Emerson, E. and Robertson, J. (in press) Review of evaluative research on case management for people with intellectual disabilities, in C. Bigby, E. Ozanne and C. Fyffe (eds) *Issues in Case Management Practice for People with Intellectual Disabilities: A Handbook for Practitioners.* London: Jessica Kingsley, pp. 280–99.

Emerson, E., Malam, S., Davies, I. and Spencer, K. (2005) *Adults with Learning Difficulties in England 2003/4.* Leeds: NHS Health and Social Care Information Centre. Available at: www.dh.gov.uk/PublicationsAndStatistics/Published-Survey/ListOfSurveySince1990/GeneralSurveys/GeneralSurveysArticle/fs/en?CONTENT_ID=4081207&chk=u%2Bd5fv

Emerson, E., Fujiura, G. and Hatton, C. (in press) International perspectives, in S. Odom, R. Horner, M. Snell and J. Blacher (eds) *Handbook on Developmental Disabilities.* New York: Guilford Press.

Greig, R. (2005) *The Story So Far . . .* London: Department of Health. Available at: www.valuingpeople.gov.uk/documents/VPReviewReportLong.pdf

Hatton, C. (2002) People with intellectual disabilities from ethnic minority communities in the US and the UK, *International Review of Research in Mental Retardation*, 25: 209–39.

Hatton, C. (2005) Poorly served. *Community Care*, 15–21 September, 36–7.

Hatton, C. (2006) Improving services for people from minority ethnic communities: the national survey returns. Paper presented at ARC National Conference on Ethnicity and Learning Disabilities, London, November.

Hatton, C., Akram, Y., Shah, R., Robertson, J. and Emerson, E. (2004a) *Supporting South Asian Families with a Child with Severe Disabilities*. London: Jessica Kingsley.

Hatton, C., Turner, S., Shah, R., Rahim, N. and Stansfield, J. (2004b) *What about Faith? Meeting the Religious Needs of People with Learning Disabilities: A Good Practice Guide*. London: Foundation for People with Learning Disabilities.

Khan, N., Rahim, N. and Routledge, M. (2004) Person centred planning and people from South Asian communities: some experiences from one locality. Available at: Valuing People Support Team website, http://valuingpeople.gov.uk/dynamic/valuingpeople88.jsp

Mir, G. and Raghavan, R. (2005) Culture and ethnicity: developing accessible and appropriate services for health and social care, in G. Grant, P. Goward, M. Richardson and P. Ramcharan (eds) *Learning Disability: A Life Cycle Approach to Valuing People*. Maidenhead: Open University Press, pp. 515–37.

Mir, G., Nocon, A. and Ahmad, W., with Jones, L. (2001) *Learning Difficulties and Ethnicity*. London: Department of Health.

Modood, T., Berthoud, R., Lakey, J., Nazroo, J., Smith, P., Virdee, S. and Beishon, S. (1997) *Ethnic Minorities in Britain: Diversity and Disadvantage*. London: Policy Studies Institute.

National Statistics Online (2003a) 2001 Census: Ethnicity population size. Available at www.statistics.gov.uk/cci/nugget.asp?id=273

National Statistics Online (2003b) 2001 Census: Religion in Britain. Available at www.statistics.gov.uk/cci/nugget.asp?id=293

National Statistics Online (2005) *2001* Census: People and Migration. Available at www.statistics.gov.uk/CCI/nugget.asp?ID=767&Pos=3&ColRank=2&Rank=224

Nazroo, J.Y. (1997) *The Health of Britain's Ethnic Minorities*. London: Policy Studies Institute.

Nazroo, J.Y. (1998) *Ethnicity and Mental Health: Findings from a National Community Survey*. London: Policy Studies Institute.

Oranu, N. (unpublished) Person centred planning in the London Borough of Hackney. Unpublished report, London Borough of Hackney.

Parmar, R., Brown, J., Shelton, C. and Potter, M. (2004) *Person Centred Planning with People from Leicester's Asian Communities*. Leicester: Leicester City Social Care and Health Department. Available at: http://valuingpeople.gov.uk/dynamic/valuingpeople88.jsp

Robertson, J., Emerson, E., Hatton, et al. (2005) *The Impact of Person Centred Planning: A Report to the Department of Health*. Lancaster: Institute for Health

Research, Lancaster University. Available at: http://www.lancs.ac.uk/fass/ihr/research/learning/projects/person.htm

Robertson, J., Emerson, E., Hatton, C., Elliott, J., McIntosh, B., Swift, P., Krijnen-Kemp, E., Towers, C., Romeo, R., Knapp, M., Sanderson, H., Routledge, M., Oakes, P. and Joyce, T. (2006) Longitudinal analysis of the impact and cost of person centered planning for people with intellectual disabilities in England. *American Journal on Mental Retardation*, 111: 400–16.

Robertson, J., Hatton, C., Emerson, E., Elliott, J., McIntosh, B., Swift, P., Krinjen-Kemp, E., Towers, C., Romeo, R., Knapp, M., Sanderson, H., Routledge, M., Oakes, P. and Joyce, T. (2007) Reported barriers to the implementation of person centred planning for people with intellectual disabilities in the UK. *Journal of Applied Research in Intellectual Disabilities*, 20: 297–307.

Sanderson, H. (2000) *Person Centred Planning: Key Features and Approaches*. York: Joseph Rowntree Foundation.

Sanderson, H., Thompson, J. and Kilbane, J. (2006) *The Emergence of Person Centred Planning as Evidence Based Practice*. Manchester: Helen Sanderson Associates, http://www.helensandersonassociates.co.uk/reading_person_09.htm

Shah, R. (2005) Addressing ethnicity and the multicultural context, in P. Cambridge and S. Carnaby (eds) *Person Centred Planning and Care Management with People with Learning Disabilities*. London: Jessica Kingsley.

Shah, R. and Hatton, C. (in press) *Learning Disabilities and Ethnicity: Getting Your Acts Together*. Manchester: Disability Rights Commission.

Triandis, H.C. (1995) *Individualism and Collectivism*. Boulder, CO: Westview Press.

Valuing People Support Team (2004) *Learning Difficulties and Ethnicity: A Framework for Action*. London: Department of Health. Available at: http://www.valuingpeople.gov.uk/EthnicityFramework.htm

Useful resources

Ethnicity Training Training (University of Leeds) www.etn.leeds.ac.uk/

The National Learning Disability and Ethnicity Network (Association for Real Change)   www.arcuk.org.uk/413/en/the+national+learning+disability+and+ethnicity+network+%28lden%29.html

Valuing People Support Team (2004) *Learning Difficulties and Ethnicity: A Framework for Action*. London: Department of Health. www.valuingpeople.gov.uk/EthnicityFramework.htm

Valuing People Support Team Ethnicity Resources web page, valuingpeople.gov.uk/dynamic/valuingpeople86.jsp

9 Person centred transition

Helen Sanderson and Chris Sholl with Linda Jordan

Key issues

- Experiences of transitions
- Legal context of transitions
- Year 9 person centred reviews
- Year 10 person centred reviews
- Transition Pathways
- Person centred approaches to transition

Introduction

Transition from school to work or college can be an exciting time of new opportunities, choices and increasing independence. It can also be a time of anxiety and confusion for young people and their families as they move from familiar people and places into 'the unknown'. For all young people it is a crucial time for thinking carefully about their life, and what they want for the future. However, all too often, planning can go on around young people without truly listening to them. In this chapter we explore people's current experiences of transition, and introduce a person centred approach of value at this point in a person's life. We focus on the Year 9 and Year 10 transition reviews and the Transition Pathway. Finally, we explore how professionals can use person centred thinking skills to help people move into adult life.

Experiences of transition

There is a growing, pretty depressing, literature on transition to adulthood for young people with learning disabilities:

- Young people with learning disabilities often receive little support to enable them to make the transition from college to employment or other meaningful activity; or from the parental home to their own home.
- Friends and sexual relationships are important issues for young people but assessments and services rarely consider these issues and can sometimes create obstacles.
- Parents report problems getting advice and information after Year 11, *'because staff from different services did not work together, or because they received conflicting advice from staff working in different services'* (Dewson et al. 2004).

It is clear that transition planning is not working for many young people. In one survey (Heslop et al. 2001) it was found that:

- Only two-thirds of young people who should have had a transitional plan had one.
- The proportion leaving school without a transitional plan increased between 1998 and 2000 (the period covered by the study).
- There were wide variations in the quality of transition planning: in some cases it was ad hoc, confused and unco-ordinated.
- Over 40 per cent of transition plans did not cover transfer to adult services at all, generally the transfer to adult social care and health services were poorly covered in transition plans.
- Lack of planning led to uncertainty and stress for families.
- There were wide discrepancies between what families wanted to be covered (information on leisure and social opportunities, benefits, future housing options and further education opportunities) and what the plans actually covered.

The experiences of people and their families in this more recent research almost exactly mirror those from a similar study 10 years ago (Hirst and Flynn 1992). In essence, the 1992 study described:

- poor co-ordination between the agencies responsible for services for children and adults, leading to dislocating experiences for young people and their families;
- lack of effective power for young people and their families within transition planning systems;
- lack of choice and opportunity on leaving school (and afterwards), for young people with learning disabilities.

This chapter argues that incorporating person centred thinking and planning into young people's everyday lives can really make a difference and help to overcome some of the difficulties outlined above. In addition, helping the professionals involved by giving them tools they can use to be more person centred could also have a real impact on their job satisfaction. Central to achieving this, however, is the premise that person centred thinking and planning in transition should not be seen as an 'add-on', rather, it should be an integral part of people's everyday lives.

Activity 9.1

Think back to when you were preparing to leave school:

- How did you decide what to do next?
- Where did you get information from?
- Who helped you?
- Are you still doing what you decided when you left education?

When one of the authors (Helen) was thinking about leaving school, her careers advisor gave her a questionnaire to complete. Based on the scores, it gave her three possible career options, one of which was a job she had never even heard of. Her results suggested working in theatre management!

She loved Art, English and Biology, so she spent some time in the library trying to work out which careers could combine all three. She secretly wanted to be a doctor, but ended up looking at Occupational Therapy, which, since she had a desire to work with people in a creative way seemed an option that might be fulfilling. She then went to visit a few Occupational Therapy departments, decided that this was for her and applied to the appropriate colleges.

In thinking about the transition from school to work the above story, and possibly your own experience, indicate the need to know three things:

- what is important to you, including your hopes and strengths;
- what is possible;
- how to make that happen locally.

What was important to Helen was working with people, and she dreamed of being a doctor. Doing the questionnaire gave her an insight into what was possible, beyond what she already knew. Finally, when she had decided on Occupational Therapy, meeting local Occupational Therapists helped her to work out what actions were necessary.

All the research and the anecdotal evidence we have indicate that young people with learning disabilities want the same thing as their non-disabled peers. Through consultation it is clear that:

[they] expect to go to work or college, have a social life, continue their hobbies, make friends and have relationships. The young people do not mention use of services in the future; but they do want very practical information and support that would enable them 'to be in charge of their lives and live more independently'.

(SCIE 2004)

However, for many young people with disabilities, transition continues to be seen as a straight progression from special school to residential college or day centre.

Activity 9.2

Write down the key differences between the experience of moving to adulthood for disabled and non-disabled young people.

Table 9.1 shows, all too often, planning can go on around young people. They may have the experience of meeting lots of different professionals who focus

Table 9.1 Comparison of actual and possible transition processes

What transition is like for most young people	*What it can be like for many young people who have additional support needs*
Lots of practice in making choices and decisions throughout childhood, ideas come from friends, school, family, marketing and other places	Few opportunities to have choices or make decisions
Information is aimed at the young person and comes from lots of sources	Information is aimed at parents, through the school and specialist services
Options are around what the person wants to do, widening choices	Assessment is by people who may not have met the person, based around what 'people like him' need
Choices are made by the young person with advice, and there can be change over time	Options are for specialist services only, based on disability and what the person cannot do
Discussion is with friends, as well as parents and school	Discussion happens in meetings, and involve professionals and parents
The young person makes the decisions	Decisions are usually made by parents
Lots of ways to get confidence	Few opportunities to build confidence
You can change your mind	You get one option to try, it feels hard to change your mind

Source: Taken from Moving on to Adult Life (2004: 35).

on what is *important for* them and not *important to* them, and who do not link up together to provide the help and support that they need.

The legal context for transition

There is a range of guidance and legislation in addition to *Valuing People* (Department of Health 2001) that can be used by statutory agencies to try and change this experience, and support the use of person centred approaches in transition planning. The following is a summary of the key guidance and legislation.

The Special Educational Needs Code of Practice (2001) requires that transition planning should be:

- *participative* – involving the young person in a meaningful way because their views and aspirations are central to the process;
- *holistic* – a young person's aspirations and needs will touch on every aspect of their future lives and hence there must be a holistic approach to planning and support;
- *supportive* – the main purpose of the statutory transition and annual review process is to support young people, their parents and the professionals who work with them in the process of making decisions about the next stage of their lives;
- *evolving* – the Year 9 review and leaving school stages are just steps in the transition of young people towards adulthood. They are part of a much longer and gradually evolving process;
- *inclusive* – as part of becoming fully inclusive, schools will need to ensure that their careers education and guidance programmes form a part of the transition planning process and meet the requirements of all pupils;
- *collaborative* – effective transition planning requires teaching staff, parents and professionals from other agencies to work closely together.

Every Child Matters and the *Children Act* (2004) set out the programme needed to deliver integrated support and services for children and young people, including five outcomes that young people say are essential to well-being in later life:

- enjoying and achieving;
- staying safe;
- being healthy;
- making a positive contribution;
- economic well-being.

The National Service Framework for Children, Young People and Maternity Services (2004) requires local authorities, Primary Care Trusts and NHS Trusts to ensure that transition planning has as its main focus the fulfilment of hopes, dreams and potential of the disabled young person. It stresses that transition planning should take a person centred approach.

Improving the Life Chances of Disabled People Cabinet Office (2005) sets out an ambitious vision for the future and has transition as one of its four priorities. Its ambition is that *'by 2025, disabled people in Britain should have full opportunities and choices to improve their quality of life and will be respected and included as equal members of society'* (2005: 43).

It identifies three key ingredients for effective support for disabled young people to ensure that they enter adulthood able to participate and be fully included:

- planning for transition focused on individual needs;
- continuous service provision;
- access to a more transparent and appropriate menu of opportunities and choices.

It indicates that *'over time, individualised budgets will allow seamless transition from childhood to adult services, providing disabled young people and their families with choice and empowerment'* and that *'personalisation in planning will require increased access to advocacy and information; person-centred planning approaches to be used widely'*. It also emphasises that the role of families needs to be recognised and supported in a way that empowers disabled young people and their parents.

The Green Paper *Independence, Wellbeing and Choice* (Department of Health 2005) supports and promotes these approaches to transition planning, recognising the importance of multi-agency co-ordination and a seamless pathway. It wants to move to a system where adults are able to take greater control of their lives. Person centred planning approaches and increased opportunities to use direct payments and individual budgets are key tools in ensuring that this vision becomes a reality, enabling people to make real choices about their lives.

The Connexions Service has a key role in helping all young people aged 13–19, and up to age 25 for young people with learning difficulties and/or disabilities, to prepare for the transition from school to adult life. The Assessment, Planning and Implementation and Review tool (APIR) used by Connexions personal advisers should ensure the involvement of young people in planning for their future lives.

Ensuring that this guidance is followed, in order that young people achieve the adult lives they want and dream about, is the challenge to us all. Person centred thinking tools and approaches in transition planning and reviews greatly assist this approach. They can be used by everyone who has an interest in or a responsibility for supporting young people in transition.

Person centred thinking and planning in transition

Valuing People (Department of Health 2001) explicitly requires that people in transition to adulthood have access to person centred planning by the year 2004. If person centred planning is to play its potentially very useful role in transition, it is important to implement it in the right context and with care. A recent reflection on the implementation of person centred planning (Routledge and Gitsham 2004) reminds us that person centred planning in itself cannot, however, be a panacea. As the Department of Health guidance stated:

> *Person centred planning ... cannot substitute for quality leadership, adequate resources efficiently used, skilled and energised staff or service development work and system changes.*
>
> (Department of Health 2001: 19)

Person centred planning is likely to work best in a context where the following conditions are found:

- good local joint systems in place to bring coherence to agency and professional transition practice;
- support for families and young people to take greater control of the design of services and supports;
- a local drive to develop wider choices at school leaving and beyond.

The Valuing People Support Team have developed a toolkit for transition champions, and this suggests ways forward in developing effective local systems and partnerships as well as in the use of person centred thinking and planning in transition. Partnership Boards have been required to develop local strategies to expand choice and control in key areas relevant to young people in transition and guidance has been developed to support these developments in, for example, day service modernisation, housing and employment.

In applying a person centred approach in transition, it is important to think about three questions:

1   What is important to the young person now and for the future, and what support do they want and need?
2   What is the best that could happen – what is possible?
3   What is practical and possible for the young person?

If we only learn what is important to the young person without knowing what is possible, then we will see the young person simply fitting in with what is available, for example, residential college or a place in the day service. We need to go further than this and learn, what is the best that can happen for young people? We then need to work together to make this happen locally.

The Year 9 person centred transition review is designed to focus on what is important to the young person, what support they need (what is important for them) and what is working and not working in their life. The Year 10 person centred transition review process takes this further by looking at what is possible (best possible examples of what other people have achieved) and prioritising which ones the young person wants to focus on.

Person centred Year 9 transition reviews

The 'Year 9' review meeting for disabled young people aged 14 plus should set the vision and a pathway to the young person's future (see Figure 9.1). However, families have not always had a good experience of these reviews. The reviews are set up and led by the school and often focus on the young person's disabilities and difficulties. With many professionals attending this meeting disabled young people and their families can find it difficult to express their views. In 2002, a different approach was tried.

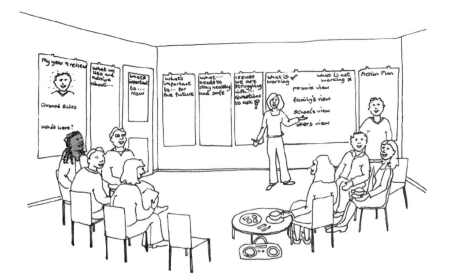

Figure 9.1 A Year 9 review meeting

The aim was to find a new process that did not require any more time or preparation yet was person centred and inclusive. The approach developed was adapted from a style of person centred planning called Essential Lifestyle Planning (Sanderson and Smull 2001). It is a powerful approach that keeps the young person at the centre, supports positive and productive review outcomes and helps people go away feeling their contribution is valued.

A person centred transition review represents a significant cultural shift for many of us. The process focuses on what matters to the young person, from their point of view. This process also explicitly recognises the contributions of the family, the school and other specialist professionals, acknowledging that the young person themselves and their families are the 'experts' on their lives and that school staff and others have specific knowledge and contributions to make.

Previously many traditional reviews and reports have begun by identifying the young person's condition and labels. This new approach turns this on its head by instead asking each member of the group what they like and admire about the young person. In this process everyone also has an opportunity to acknowledge and celebrate what is working well for the young person and their role and contribution to this. This again represents a change, as often contact between school and family is focused on what is difficult and not going well.

What is not going well is also addressed in this process, and results in jointly agreed actions. A person centred review meeting normally lasts around an hour and a half. In this time information that can be developed into a person centred plan is gathered and recorded. In this section we will describe how you can use this information to build a person centred plan, which can be the foundation of the transition process. Over the next few years, the person centred plan can be developed and reviewed, and used to enable the young person to embark on adult life.

Person centred transition reviews can be facilitated by school staff, person centred planning facilitators, professionals, family mentors or Connexions staff. Person centred review facilitators require training in person centred reviews, structured practice with coaching and regular opportunities to reflect and problem solve with others doing this work.

The aim of the Year 9 person centred review is to do the following:

1   Identify and discuss what people like and admire about the person, what is important to the person (now and for the future) and what help and support the person needs.
2   Identify and discuss what is working and not working from different people's perspectives (the person, family, school staff and others).
3   Produce and agree actions that will:

(a) support the person to get what is important to them now and in the future;
(b) maintain what is working and change what is not working;
(c) build on the person centred information and develop the information into a person centred plan.

The Year 9 person centred transition review was designed to be done with very little preparation – just ensuring that people knew what to expect and ensuring that we had done what we could to make sure that the young person was comfortable and could participate as fully as possible. However, more preparation can make it a better experience for everyone, and over the last two years there have been many creative ways that facilitators and schools have helped people and families to prepare. In one area, they even made the young person a jigsaw of the headings of the review! Many forward-thinking schools are now integrating preparing for the Year 9 review into their curriculum.

> *This is much better, at the old reviews people just told you what they thought. I have had to face my worries for Sarah in the future today, but I have felt very supported and positive, the last review was insignificant compared to this one.*

(Sarah's mum)

> *They were the best Year 9 transition reviews we have attended in years . . . We felt a clear breakthrough had been achieved in transition planning. This style is the way forward.*

(Deputy Head)

> *I enjoyed hearing what people had to say about me.*

(Young person)

Person centred Year 10 transition reviews

As suggested earlier, for a successful transition we need to know what is important to the young person, what is possible, and then how to make this happen. The Year 10 review (see Figure 9.2) builds on the information and actions developed in the Year 9 review and looks at what is possible for the young person, and how to make this happen.

The aim of the Year 10 person centred review is to do the following:

1   Identify and discuss what is possible (national best practice) using the keys to citizenship as a framework.
2   Look at what is practical and possible locally and prioritise what to focus on now.

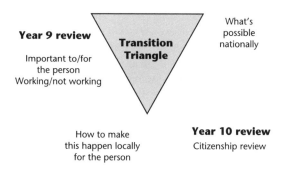

Figure 9.2   The transition triangle

3   Agree actions that will take the young person closer to what is practical and possible, taking into account what is important to them and what support they need.

Jennie's mum, Suzi, describes Jennie's Year 10 review (see Box 9.1):

Box 9.1 Jennie's transition review

This transition review was arranged to specifically look at Jennie's immediate and long-term future and how everyone could work together to ensure this happened as smoothly as possible for Jennie. It was structured around three questions: (1) What is possible for Jennie's future? (2) What do we want for Jennie's future? and (3) What are we going to do to move this forward?

Helen facilitated the review. We started by introducing ourselves and who we are in Jennie's life, and then we checked what we had done regarding the actions we had set from the previous review. The review was very well attended and included family, friends, support workers, teacher, speech therapist, Connexions, social worker, team leader and manager.

After the introductions Helen talked about the purpose of the meeting and introduced us to Keys to Citizenship. She used a large chart and explained each key for the group to consider when thinking about what could be possible and positive for Jennie's future. Helen went through the six keys: self-determination, direction, money, home, support and community life, and talked about what was practical and possible (and best practice) for each key. Helen then asked the group if they had any questions. No one said anything – I think everyone was still taking the information in!

There were blank pieces of flip chart paper for each key on the wall. We each had a marker pen and we thought about the ideas from the Keys chart, and wrote the ones that we would like to see in Jennie's future on the flip chart paper.

Some of us thought about questions then, and Helen answered these as we were writing. We looked at what everyone had written. Helen drew around the major themes that people had written about, so that we could see three or four clear areas for each key. Then she gave us all three sticky dots and asked us to put them on the areas that we wanted to start working on now. After we had placed our dots and sat down, Helen counted the dots and gave each one a 'score'. We then started to work through each one, highest score first, and agreed on actions that we wanted to take.

Some of the actions that came from Jennie's review were:

- increasing leisure opportunities;
- looking at 16+ education;
- forming a circle of support;
- thinking about future living arrangements.

We ended the meeting by each saying something that we had appreciated about our time together, and setting a date for a follow-up meeting.

People said the meeting had been:

'A really good opportunity for everyone to work together for Jennie's future', 'Good to meet others working with and supporting Jennie', 'A really positive review', 'Wish this could happen for all the children I work with.'

I remember looking at everyone writing on the sheets of paper and jointly deciding what we should concentrate on to help Jennie. It was a really nice feeling knowing that I wasn't on my own and people were happy and willing to support Jennie and her planning process.

This was Jennie's second Person Centred Planning review. She had her first person centred review last year, where people came together to think about what is important to Jennie, and what support she wants and needs. As Jennie's mum, I was keen that we should look at the actions we had agreed then, and begin to think about her future. The group of people invited to her Year 9 review had already had a taste of these new ways of planning and meeting together. The information from the last review is now part of Jennie's Essential Lifestyle Plan.[1] It was also really important that Jennie can start to be involved in planning for her future.

A person centred Transition Pathway

The Transition Pathway integrates the Year 9 and the Year 10 person centred transition reviews into a pathway process. It was produced as a response to a consultation with young people, their families and a range of professionals in nine local authorities in the West Midlands. By listening to young people and their families' stories about what was important to them in transition, as well as asking professionals about what would help improve person centred transition planning, a multi-agency team developed the Transition Pathway (Sholl et al. 2005).

The Transition Pathway is a pack of accessible guidance and tools which can be used by anyone with an interest in supporting young people (age 13–25) in the transition to adult life. It provides a firm foundation to person centred transition planning.

From 2003 to 2005, more than 100 young disabled people and their families, professionals and staff took part in the West Midlands Transition Pathway project. There was wide consultation about what was important to young people in planning for their adult lives, what good things are happening, and what needs to change. Many young people felt that they were not listened to and the things that were important to them were not discussed in transition planning. Many families felt that they did not know enough about the transition process, and how they could get advice and support. Many professionals felt uncertain about their own and other professionals' roles in transition planning. In order to address these issues, draft guidance was produced by a multi-agency working group which included young people and family carers.

This guidance was then tested out by over 100 young people in a range of settings and their feedback and suggestions were used to help develop the final products. There was also ongoing consultation with families and a wide range of professionals who were involved with the young people to find out what they needed to help improve transition and to ensure young people have the adult lives they want and dream about.

The result of this collaboration is the Transition Pathway guidance and tools to support person centred transition planning and The Big Picture guide to transition for young people aged 13–25 (Sholl et al. 2005): www.transitionpathway.co.uk

The Transition Pathway is based upon a process map which divides the transition process into five stages. The stages incorporate the Year 9 and the Year 10 reviews and are:

Stage 1 – Getting Ready
Stage 2 – Making the Transition Plan
Stage 3 – Planning Ahead
Stage 4 – Leaving School
Stage 5 – Moving On.

For each stage it is specified what the law and government guidance says and what should happen. The Year 9 person centred transition review takes place in Stage 2, and the Year 10 person centred transition review in Stage 3.

The Transition Pathway pack is now available for use anywhere. It can be used by anyone with an interest in transition to have a better understanding of their own and other people's roles and responsibilities in transition planning. The tools can be used to help them listen to young people and support them to get the lives they want and dream for. Some of the ways the Transition Pathway tools can be used are as follows:

- They have been incorporated into the curriculum.
- To help young people prepare for their transition review.
- In conjunction with person centred transition reviews.
- Some young people have used the tools to help them organise their own reviews and planning meetings.
- Some young people have developed their own 'My Life, My Future' personal workbooks, linked to The Big Picture and the planning tools (see Box 9.2).

Box 9.2 Sammie's story: how she used the Transition Pathway, The Big Picture and her person centred review

Sammie is 13 and lives with her mum and brother. She is in Year 9 of a special school for students with learning disabilities. Sammie helped the Transition Pathway project and the person centred review project to find out more about how they link together to support person centred transition planning. The Transition Pathway for Sammie followed the five stages of the transition process.

1 Getting ready for the transition review

In school, Sammie and her classmates used The Big Picture to help them think about what is important to them now and who can help them plan for the future.

Sammie's teacher used The Big Picture as part of the school curriculum. This helped Sammie to think about some of the things that were important to her. This included things like having friends, doing as much as she can for herself, and having lots of things to do. Sammie used photos and pictures to develop her own 'My Life, My Future' book which she uses to show other people what is important to her.

Sammie's school was also taking part in the person centred transition review project. As part of the project, Kate and Diane were training to be independent facilitators. They met Sammie at school and she showed them her 'My Life, My Future' book. This helped them to get to know Sammie and the sort of things that she liked doing, new things she'd like to do and things she needs help with.

Kate and Diane also visited Sammie and her family at home. They gave Sammie's mum and brother The Big Picture and the Getting Ready sheets from the Transition Pathway pack to help them prepare for the person centred transition review.

They all spent time out in the garden. Sammie enjoyed showing them how she could bounce on the trampoline. Kate took Sammie's photo on the trampoline and a photo of her dog Flash so she could take them to her review. Sammie showed Kate and Diane her CDs and chose a Kylie CD to play at her review meeting.

Doing this preparation and gathering this information really helped Sammie and her family to think about what they would like to talk about at the review.

2 Making the Transition Plan – at the person centred transition review

Sammie chose the people who came to her review. Everyone wrote on the flip chart sheets about Sammie (see Figure 9.3).

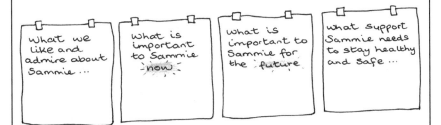

Figure 9.3   Sammie's flip charts

Sammie used her 'My Life, My Future' book and the photos Kate had taken to show people what was important to her.

Holding the review in this way gave Sammie the opportunity to share what was important to her now and for the future in ways that were appropriate to her. It gave other people there a full picture of Sammie. People who were there said things like, 'It brought a lot of honesty to the meeting'; 'It was good to have prepared before the meeting'; 'I feel that I know Sammie the person.'

A transition plan and action plan were produced at the meeting, saying what needed to happen, who would do this and when. This included things like finding out about a gym club, trying out a new communication aid and doing travel training.

3 Planning ahead

Sammie will continue using The Big Picture and her 'My Life, My Future' book to carry on planning and recording what is important to her. She will use these to help her prepare for and share information at her next review meeting in Year 10 at school.

Sammie's family has started thinking about the future in a way that feels supported. They have made links with key people who can support transition planning with Sammie, and feel more positive about the future. Sammie's mum says, '*It feels less scary.*' They will continue to use the guidance in the Transition Pathway to help them think about the future and different things that Sammie can do. At the next review in Year 10, they will learn more about other opportunities like Direct Payments and in Control.

4 Leaving school

As the time approaches for Sammie to leave school, she will continue using The Big Picture to help with more detailed planning about what she wants to do when she leaves school. She will start visiting different places, so she has a better idea of what they are like. She will take her 'My Life, My Future' book with her to show new people she meets what is important to her. It can also be used to help people to do any assessments she needs, for example, for an individualised budget.

5 Moving On

Sammie lives in an area which, at the time of writing, was developing self-directed support and individual budgets with a specific focus on young people in transition. By starting to plan early at Sammie's transition review, and continuing to plan in a person centred way, Sammie will have more choice in and control over the adult life she hopes and dreams for.

- They have used the 'My Life, My Future' personal workbooks to share information with new people in their lives and to provide information for assessments.
- Families have used the Transition Pathway to help them understand what should happen and when.
- The Transition Pathway transition plan format has replaced previous formats.

The Transition Pathway is designed to ensure that young people, and what is most important to them, are central to the transition planning process. For instance, many young people say that having fun and keeping in touch with friends is very important to them, but things like that are very rarely discussed in transition meetings.

The Transition Pathway and The Big Picture are being used in many schools and local authority areas. The tools can be used to support other processes, for example, person centred transition reviews and planning for 'in Control' individualised budgets.

Using person centred thinking skills in transition

Many forward-thinking schools are already using a person centred approach and person centred thinking tools can be useful additions to their practice, particularly as they can be adapted for use within the curriculum.

The Year 9 person centred review process is based on three person centred thinking skills: (1) 'like and admire'; (2) 'important to and support to stay healthy and safe'; and (3) 'working/not working from different perspectives'. This next section will demonstrate that there are also a range of different ways in which the same skills can be used to good effect and will discuss the interface of these approaches with the Year 9 and Year 10 reviews. These include examples such as Laura's one-page plan, Ellie's one-page plan (see Box 9.4), and Julie's 9–3.15 plan (see Box 9.5).

One of the ways to use what is important to and for a child or young person is to record this as a 'living description'. This can be done on one page – as a one-page profile or in more detail. More detailed plans could cover all of the young person's life, or for a specific time period, for example, the time that they are at school. Julie has a 9–3.15 plan because this is the time that she spends at school (see Box 9.5). These plans can be used as preparation for transition, or can develop from the information gathered at a person centred Year 9 review.

In Laura's one-page profile there is information about what people like and admire about her (and what she likes about herself), what is important to her, and what is important for her (phrased as 'how to support Laura') (see Box 9.3). Laura's one-page profile simply focused on what people like and admired about Laura and what she is good at.

Box 9.3 Laura's one-page profile

Laura's mum described how she developed a one-page profile for her daughter.

> My daughter, Laura, had started to say that she did not want to go to school and that she was scared of her teacher. She had been told off for not having the right clothes for sports at school. We went to meet the teacher, who said that she had not really been able to get to know Laura as she is quiet in class. She had not told Laura off about clothes for sports, but had pointed out that if she only had shorts to wear rather than jogging bottoms, then her legs would get cold.

We decided that we needed to help the teacher to learn about Laura quickly, and that we had some information about how to support Laura that could be helpful.

We talked to Laura and got some ideas together in a draft profile. Over Christmas, when we were with our extended family, Laura showed the profile to each individual family member and they added their information. It was lovely for Laura to hear what her family likes and admires about her (see Figure 9.4). Then, after Christmas, over a hot chocolate in a café, Laura and I thought about what information to keep in and what to leave out.

Laura and I shared it with the teacher after school whose response was '*This would have been very useful to have had at the beginning of the year.*' She talked about how helpful this information would be at some of the important transition times, like children coming from nursery into school, and moving from Key Stage 1 to Key Stage 2, moving on to secondary school or preparing for transition. She was, however, concerned that one-page profiles did not become an additional expectation on overworked teachers!

Laura is now about to move into her next class. We moved the text from her profile to one side to create some space for recording changes in Laura's life. Laura wrote about her stick insect eggs hatching. Her friend wrote that she is 'good to trust'. We gave it to her teacher, who added her comments, and then I made these changes to the profile. Laura did not want to draw a picture of herself this time, she wanted a photo instead.

Laura's profile was shared with her next teacher, who commented:

'*It was great to get a fuller picture of who Laura is – her likes and dislikes and her character. This will be really useful for me to get to know Laura.*'

One of our dreams is for all children to have their own person centred plans, in all mainstream and special schools. Closer to reality, however, teachers would not be able to read, use and add to very detailed person centred plans on all children in their class. We thought that a one-page profile (see Figure 9.4) would give a snapshot of Laura, which would enable her teacher to ask Laura whether her stick insects eggs had hatched yet, talk about her profiles for her birthday party and what she enjoyed about going to Oasis with her family. Equally important, she would know that Laura will perceive a small negative comment as a big telling off, and needs a lot of encouragement and support.

In services for children with disabilities, Year 9 person centred transition reviews gather information that can be used to develop a one-page or a more detailed profile. Where children already have a one-page profile, the person centred transition reviews could build on this information.

We must be very clear about the purpose of a one-page profile – it is to provide an insight into part of someone's life in a specific context. The key is purpose and context. The teacher does not need to know all the nuances of Laura's morning routine, etc., but does need to know how best to support Laura in class, and have a head start in getting to know her.

Laura

What others like about me, and what I like about myself

Artistic, Caring, Good at climbing, swimming and sports,
Gives great cuddles, Creative, Good at making, drawing and building stuff,
Great at reading, Trustworthy, Thoughtful, Adventurous, Totally reliable

What is important to me

- My cats Jess and Mia
- Playing with my friends – Eleanor, Rebecca, Abi, Emily, Caitlin, Freya, Kate, Olivia and Freya FB
- Seeing my cousins, Honor, Phoebe, Maya, Tyler and Joshua
- Going to Centre Parcs every year with Granny, Aunty Wendy, Uncle Dave, Aunty Clare and Uncle Miguel
- My Moose who sleeps on my bed
- Knowing what is going to happen each day, and planning ahead for special things like my birthday (I like to plan my party about 4 months in advance!)
- Being helpful in class
- Knowing what is being asked of me in class
- Supporting Manchester City and going to matches with Gill and Babs

How to support Laura

- Laura is sensitive and perceives a small negative comment as a big telling off. A non confrontational approach works best with Laura
- Laura needs lots of praise and encouragement
- Laura does not like change very much and particularly needs lots of reassurance about changing classes
- Laura can seem quiet and shy before you get to know her but she is confident enough to initiate a conversation with a teacher or adult

Thank you to Mrs Hardman, Mrs. Stephenson, Granny, Aunty Wendy, Uncle Dave, Aunty Clare, Uncle Miguel, Honor, Uncle Ju, and Aunty Nikki for helping Laura, Mummy and Daddy to write Laura's plan for school January 2007

Figure 9.4   Laura's one-page profile

In Year 10 reviews, we ask people about what is important to them now and for the future. This could be one way of capturing this information and sharing it in the review, or recording the information from the review.

Box 9.4 Ellie's one-page 'future' profile

Laura's one-page profile uses the person centred thinking tools 'important to' and 'important for'. Ellie's one-page profile just captures what is important to her now, and for the future (see Figure 9.5). Ellie is in Year 7. She has been thinking about her future, and has recorded this as a one-page profile that says what people like and admire about her, what is important to her, and what is important to her for the future. She likes using clip art on the computer, and used this to illustrate her profile. She talks to her mum about what she wants to do in the future, and as things change, she will change her profile. Her mum says it is a good way to think with Ellie about what she is enjoying at the moment, and how her profiles for the future build on who she is (what others like and admire about her) and what matters to her (what is important to her now). Ellie says she will use this when she is thinking about choosing her options at school.

Conclusion

The Transition Pathway and the Year 9 and Year 10 reviews provide a framework for delivering a person centred approach to transition. The person centred thinking tools that have been used to create the one-page profiles, and to implement Julie's 9–3.15 plan, offer professionals examples of ways to develop their practices with young people in transition. We hope that people use these processes to help young people to discover and create the futures that they want. We expect that this will lead to fewer and fewer people going into traditional day services, and instead, young people having paid work, having their own individual budgets or direct payments, employing their own staff, enjoying full lives and being contributing members of their communities. When we have achieved this for people moving from adolescence to adulthood, then hopefully the transition experience will have significantly improved for people and their families.

Note

1   To see Jennie's plan, go to www.helensandersonassociates.co.uk

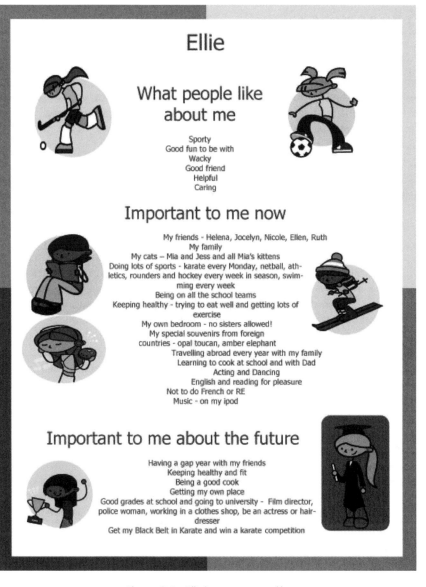

Ellie

What people like about me

Sporty
Good fun to be with
Wacky
Good friend
Helpful
Caring

Important to me now

My friends - Helena, Jocelyn, Nicole, Ellen, Ruth
My family
My cats – Mia and Jess and all Mia's kittens
Doing lots of sports - karate every Monday, netball, athletics, rounders and hockey every week in season, swimming every week
Being on all the school teams
Keeping healthy - trying to eat well and getting lots of exercise
My own bedroom - no sisters allowed!
My special souvenirs from foreign countries - opal toucan, amber elephant
Travelling abroad every year with my family
Learning to cook at school and with Dad
Acting and Dancing
English and reading for pleasure
Not to do French or RE
Music - on my ipod

Important to me about the future

Having a gap year with my friends
Keeping healthy and fit
Being a good cook
Getting my own place
Good grades at school and going to university - Film director, police woman, working in a clothes shop, be an actress or hairdresser
Get my Black Belt in Karate and win a karate competition

Figure 9.5   Ellie's one-page profile

Box 9.5 Julie's 9–3.15 plan

Julie attends a mainstream school. She is a popular, sunny and determined girl. She has Down's syndrome and an exotic collection of other health-related labels. Her mum had been frustrated with the support that she had been receiving at school, and talked about this to another mum. Together they approached the head teacher and explored the idea of developing a 9–3.15 plan for Julie that describes who Julie is, what is important to her, and the support she needs at school.

They used her Individual Education Plan and records from the school in order to start developing the plan, and then they added information from the family. The SENCO, her teacher, and Julie's learning support assistants added their information too. The plan now has up-to-date information to help everyone supporting Julie to share what they are learning about Julie and to have a living record of who she is and how best to support her at school. The SENCO is exploring whether this plan could replace the existing Individual Education Format.

In Julie's 9–3.15 plan it describes what is important to and for her while she is at school. This was important as one of the difficulties had been that her learning support assistants had been seeing some of their core responsibilities as areas where they had creativity and judgement. This particularly refers to the fact that it is important for Julie that she is not taught using phonics, but by using another approach which works better for her. Her support assistants in school had been trying different ways to teach her phonics, rather than following the clear guidelines about the approach that should be used. Essentially therefore this was not a creativity and judgement issue for them, it was a core responsibility to use the agreed approach. When Julie's 9–3.15 plan had been agreed, the doughnut was used to clarify roles and responsibilities in relation to putting the plan into practice. This included what the family, head teacher, her teacher, SENCO and learning support assistants were responsible for. In particular, it was important to identify what and where individuals could use creativity and judgement.

As part of Julie's 9–3.15 plan the family and teacher will be using the matching staff form to think about the best person to support Julie in her new class. They will use this to either see which of the four learning support assistants would be the best fit for Julie or if they need to consider recruiting someone just for Julie at some point in the future.

Julie's learning support assistant fills in a diary for Julie everyday. It describes the subjects that she has been doing. Mum and the teacher want to try to adapt the learning log for the learning support assistant to fill in instead, so that it captures more of what we are learning about Julie, instead of just recording what she did. Mum and the teacher plan to look at the learning logs together for half an hour every two months, to see what they tell us about Julie, and what they therefore need to change in Julie's 9–3.15 plan. Julie's plan is being used to help her prepare for her transition.

To see Julie's 9–3.15 plan, go to www.helensandersonassociates.co.uk

Annotated bibliography

Sanderson, H., Mathiesen, R. and Sweeney, C. (2007) *Person Centred Reviews* (in press). Manchester: HSA Press.
This practical visual book describes three types of person centred reviews that can be used in schools and in adult services.

Sholl, C., Dancyger, F., Dale, C. and Parsons, M. (2005) *Transition Pathway Pack*. www.transitionpathway.co.uk
The Transition Pathway is a resource pack which can be used by anybody who is involved in supporting a young person in transition to adult life. It gives information and guidance about transition and provides tools, using person centred approaches, to help young people think about, plan and lead the lives they want. The Transition Pathway Pack was also runner-up for a national award in December 2006 'Books for Teaching and Learning', sponsored by Times Educational Supplement and NASEN (National Association for Special Educational Needs).

References

Cabinet Office (2005) *Improving the Life Chances of Disabled People*. London: Stationery Office.

Department for Education and Skills (2001) *Special Educational Needs (SEN) Code of Practice*. London: DfES.

Department of Health (2001) *Valuing People: A New Strategy for Learning Disability for the 21st Century*. London: Department of Health.

Department of Health (2004) *The National Service Framework for Children, Young People and Maternity Services*. London: Department of Health.

Department of Health (2005) *Independence, Well-being and Choice. Our Vision for the Future of Social Care for Adults in England*. London: Department of Health.

Dewson, S., Aston, J., Bates, P., Ritchie, H. and Dyson, A. (2004) *Post-16 Transitions: A Longitudinal Study of Young People with Special Educational Needs: Wave Two*. DfES Research Report. London: DfES.

Heslop, P., Mallett, R., Simons, K. and Ward, L. (2001) *Bridging the Divide: The Experiences of Young People with Learning Difficulties and Their Families at Transition*. Kidderminster: BILD Publications.

Hirst, M. and Flynn, M. (1992) *This Year, Next Year, Sometime . . .? Learning Disability and Adulthood*. London: National Development Team.

Moving on to Adult Life (2004) *A Resource Pack Written for Families by Families*. Glasgow: Outside the Box.

Routledge, M. and Gitsham, N. (2004) 'Putting person centred planning in its proper place?', *Learning Disability Review*, 9(3): 21–6.

Sanderson, H., Mathiesen, R. and Sweeney, C. (2007) *Person Centred Reviews* (in press). Manchester: HSA Press.

SCIE (2004) *Involving Service Users and Carers in Social Work Education.* Resource Guide No. 2. London: Social Care Institute for Excellence.

Sholl, C., Dancyger, F., Dale, C. and Parsons, M. (2005) *Transition Pathway Pack.* www.transitionpathway.co.uk

Smull, M. and Sanderson, H. (2001) *Essential Lifestyle Planning for Everyone.* Manchester: HSA Press.

Useful resources

Department of Health
www.dh.gov.uk

Helen Sanderson Associates
www.helensandersonassociates.co.uk

Transition Pathway
www.transitionpathway.co.uk

10 People with learning disabilities planning for themselves

Julie Lunt, Jonathon Bassett, Liz Evans and Leah Jones

Key issues

- Supporting people who have a learning disability to lead their own plans
- Self-determination
- Keeping people at the centre of their plan
- Supporting other people who have a learning disability to plan
- Training people to facilitate plans
- The things that help people plan

The phrase 'person centred planning' in itself tells us that if planning is done properly people with learning disabilities are leading their own plans. They may be leading their own plan in a wide range of ways with different kinds of support. In addition, they may be training or advising others how to plan. This chapter talks about the different ways in which people can lead person centred planning and the authors use examples from their own lives and experiences to illustrate the different ways. It gives guidance on the support that people might need to be able to lead planning and describes a range of tools that can be used to support the planning process. Some of these tools are also described in other chapters of this book (see Chapters 4 and 7). This chapter also talks about people leading person centred planning and people with learning disabilities being empowered and empowering others to take control of their lives and making informed choices. Finally, it also discusses the role that professionals can have in supporting people to lead their own plans.

Jonathon, Liz and Leah are all experienced self-advocates. They are actively involved in advocacy organisations that encourage people with learning disabilities to have more control in their own lives. Supporting people in developing person centred plans and teaching people how to plan is a part of the work they do.

Professionals' involvement in supporting people with learning disabilities to lead their own plans

Professionals whose job is to make sure people with learning disabilities get support, money and health care, to help them to get the lives they want, have an important part to play in person centred planning. There are four areas where they can give their support to people with learning disabilities who are leading their own person centred plans: (1) introducing; (2) contributing; (3) safeguarding; and (4) integrating (see Figure 10.1).

Introducing

There are still people with learning disabilities and their families who do not know about person centred planning. The professional can tell these people what a plan is and help them to think about, if they want their own plan, and how they would like to be involved. To be able to do this the professional needs to do the following:

- Know what person centred planning is.
- Understand the different types of planning and be able to explain them, so the person can choose the best way for them to plan.

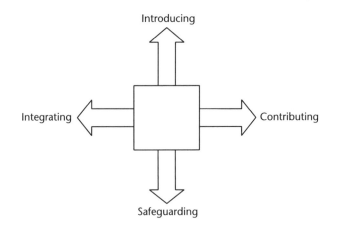

Figure 10.1   Four areas of support
Source: Kilbane and Sanderson (2005)

- Know about the information and resources that are available to help the person and their family, for example, 'Families leading planning packs' and 'Listen to me' manuals.
- Know what courses are available for people to learn about leading their own plans.
- Know who to contact to help them to plan if they would like support, for example, person centred planning co-ordinators.

Contributing

This chapter is about people leading their own plans and we will talk about the different ways people can do this later in the chapter but professionals may still make a contribution. How they do this will depend on the way in which the person wishes to lead their own plan.

The professional can:

- Facilitate the plan.
- Be part of the planning meetings.
- Help but not be part of the meeting.
- Be involved in achieving the actions on the action plan.

When professionals are supporting someone to lead their own plans they need to have good training in person centred planning. They must make sure that they understand clearly how the person wishes to be supported and what materials and information may help, such as *Our Plan for Planning*, which was written by Manchester and Liverpool People First Groups, about the support they want to stay in control of their meetings. Supporting people in leading their own plans may mean that professionals have to work evenings and weekends to attend meetings.

Safeguarding

Professionals still have a role in making sure that plans are good quality. This does not mean telling people that they are doing things wrong but means using their own experience and training to support the person to make sure all the important parts of the plan are included. This could include making sure that there is an action plan and everyone is working on achieving their actions or, if the person has chosen to have an essential Lifestyle Plan, that the detail is clear enough for everyone to understand what is important in the person's life and how they should support them.

Professionals need to be aware of the quality processes used in their area and share that information with people leading their own plans. They also need to keep up to date with new information and share this with people leading plans in a way that is meaningful to them.

Integrating

Integration means 'all the parts of the machine fit together so that it works properly and everyone uses it all the time'. With a person centred plan this means that the plan is clear with the right detail so that it is fully followed through and that it becomes fixed in everyone's mind that this is what should happen. Jackie Kilbane and Helen Sanderson, who first talked about the different ways that professionals could support person centred planning, tell us that there are three ways to integrate person centred planning into the work of the professional.

1   On an individual level, between the person, the professionals and the other people in the person's life.
2   Making sure what people learn about planning is shared with local implementation groups and people who are measuring quality and others whose job it is to collect and share information.
3   Making sure person centred approaches are always used because it has become a habit and what people learn about person centred planning is shared as it is also a habit.

Activity 10.1

How can you help integrate person centred planning and person centred approaches into your work with people who have a learning disability?

Jackie and Helen say that to be involved in integrating person centred planning professionals should do the following:

- Practise introducing, contributing and safeguarding person centred planning approaches.
- Agree with the person the best ways to include the important parts of their professional work in the plan.
- Make sure what has been learned about person centred planning is given to local implementation groups and professional groups using the methods decided by the local organisations.
- Create ways of sharing learning with other people who are involved in planning.
- Understand how person centred planning approaches can change the way professionals work, for example, in developing the training of professionals.

Whatever way professionals can support people, the key goal when planning is to support the person to take control of their own life.

Self-determination

Simon Duffy (2006) says self-determination is the first key to becoming a citizen. It is a complicated word and it is becoming another common jargon phrase used by professionals and others when they are talking about the lives of people with learning disabilities. It means 'being in charge of your own life'. Many people with learning disabilities do not have self-determination. In legal terms they are described as not having mental capacity. This means not having the ability to understand the nature and consequences of a particular decision. For example, if a person needed treatment for cancer, they would have capacity if they understood what cancer was and what might happen if they chose whether or not to have the treatment. It is often difficult to define who does have mental capacity. The law tells us we should assume someone has capacity unless we have good reason to suspect that they do not. Having a learning disability in itself is not a good enough reason.

In 2007, the new Mental Capacity Bill became law. It attempts to clarify some of the difficulties over who does and does not have capacity and how people who are considered not to have capacity should be included in decision-making processes that are about them. The decision-making agreement described later in this chapter is an example of how people can be supported. Hillary Brown, who has done a lot of work on sexuality and keeping people safe, has said that if people with learning disabilities have good information and education in a way that they can understand, then their ability to make informed decisions improves, which may give them capacity to make a decision.

When considering whether someone has capacity it is helpful to think about each decision separately. Others must not assume that because someone does not understand about cancer, they would not be able to control their money. However, there are lots of areas where people are denied opportunities to make decisions because people think that they do not have capacity. These include:

- the right to vote;
- choosing medical treatment;
- having a sexual relationship or getting married;
- being in charge of their money or getting a bank account;
- getting a job;
- having legal responsibilities;

- entering into a contract;
- having a home tenancy or a mortgage.

Even if someone may not understand the nature or consequences of something, it should not mean they cannot achieve self-determination. It does, however, require that the people around that person, including families and professionals, recognise that the person has the right to self-determination. They need to listen carefully to the person in the widest sense by hearing and responding to what the person does as well as what they say. Later in this chapter we describe how to do this.

To be listened to, and having what we think, say, or do, respected is essential for our self-esteem. It makes us feel valued and worthwhile as a citizen. Being in charge of our own lives gives us the right to make bad decisions or decisions that we later regret. We are responsible for the decision we make but in doing so we learn and develop our character. Professionals have often said to Julie, '*But we have a duty of care to keep people healthy and safe.*' This is true but this does not mean that we ignore what makes sense to someone just to keep them safe. Doing so would ignore their right to self-determination.

The 'Important to/Important for' tool developed by the Essential Lifestyles Planning Learning Community describes how to make decisions with someone which help keep them healthy and safe as well as recognising what is important to them. Julie and Jonathon have described parts of their own lives to demonstrate how it may be used.

'Important to' and 'important for'

Important to are those things which make us happy and fulfilled. What matters in how we live our life is very individual. For Jonathon, this is being in touch with his family and friends every week and to see his grandparents most weekends. He goes out with them and particularly likes to go for a meal. Going walking in the Lake District is also important. Every year Jonathon and his family go to Castleton to see the lights. He says, '*If these things didn't happen, I would NOT be very happy. I like being around my Nan and going up to my Mum's in Wales.*'

It is *important to* Julie to have enough time to get ready in the morning. This means getting up an hour before she needs to leave for work. If she is leaving early, it is important that all her clothes are laid out the night before so she can put them on straight away, also her work bags are packed and in the car. If she does not have enough time in the mornings to get ready she becomes stressed and often forgets things. This can upset her for the rest of the day.

These are the things which are *important to* us. It does not matter what other people think about them. On the other hand, what is *important for* are the things in all of our lives which need to be there to keep us healthy or safe.

We also need support from the people around us who may advise us about looking after ourselves. These are *important for* us. It is important for Jonathon to take his medicine for acne every night before bed. He says, *'If I didn't take it, I would be all spotty again and that is not nice.'* It is *important for* Julie to be able to tell her friends and family when she is having a bad time. She says, *'I need to talk about what's worrying me otherwise I dwell on it. My friends don't have to advise me. I just need to know they understand.'*

We all need a balance between what is *important to* us and what is *important for* us. We should only provide the *important for* things in a way which makes sense according to what is *important to* the person. Jonathon says, *'I love to buy computer games but it is important for me to wait until they come down in price so I can afford it.'* Staff support him with this by helping him manage his money. In this way the staff are paying attention to what is *important to* him, which is buying computer games. They believe that Jonathon could get into debt if he bought as many games as he would like. Therefore it is *important for* him that they advise and support him to understand how much money he has and how he can save to buy the games. They know that buying games is more *important to* him than buying other things.

Julie says, *'Chocolate is important to me as I enjoy eating it. It is also important to look good in my clothes. If I put on too much weight my clothes don't fit and I feel unhappy. It is important for me to watch how much chocolate I eat. I balance my love of chocolate and not getting too fat by eating chocolate only a couple of times a week. When I do, I buy my favourite which is Green and Blacks Almond bar.'* Julie has recognised that to be happy and healthy she needs to pay attention to what is *important to* and *for* her. She has made a personal decision to limit how much chocolate she eats but does not cut it out altogether. In choosing to eat her favourite bar she makes doing something that is important to her even more special.

Professionals need to listen to the person or others who know them well to find out what is important to the people they are supporting. If they have an Essential Lifestyle Plan which they are willing to share, the professional can learn from the plan how to make sure that they are making the right decisions to keep that person healthy and safe. The professional may get the best answers by chatting to the person in everyday conversations rather than by asking the question, *'What is important to you?'* They need to avoid questions that need only a yes or no answer, for example, do you like bowling? Or have a built-in answer, for example, wouldn't you like to live in a new house?

Activity 10.2

What questions do you ask to find out what is *important to* and *important for* a person you are working with?

Possible questions to ask might be:

- What makes a really good day for you?
- What makes you laugh?
- What makes you angry?
- If you could have a magic wand to make a wish come true, what would it be?
- What do you like doing on holiday or your birthday?
- What would the best support be like for you?
- If your house was burning down, what would you want to save?

How people with learning disabilities can lead their own plans

There are many different ways people who have a learning disability can and do lead their own plans.

Activity 10.3
How do you think people who have a learning disability can lead their own plans?

This can happen in the following ways:

- Keeping people at the centre of their plan.
- People leading their own plan with support.
- People leading their own plans.
- Supporting other people to lead their own plans.
- Training people in person centred planning.

Each of these allows the person who has a learning disability to take active control over their own plan and thus their own life or to support someone else who has a learning disability to do the same. We will look at each of these in more detail in the next section.

Keeping people at the centre of their plan

Listening carefully to the person who is developing a plan is the first stage in someone leading a plan, as it keeps them at the centre of the process. The person who is developing a plan may not use words to communicate or they may find it difficult to make sense of the world around them. However, if we are 'listening' to them carefully, not by hearing what they say but by observing closely what they do, we can 'hear' what is important to and for them. Our behaviour is a very powerful way of communicating how we feel. It can be more powerful than what we say as we often guard the words we use but what we do is more instinctive.

When working with someone who does not use words to communicate or has difficulties expressing themselves, the person who is supporting them to plan may ask people who know and love them what they do in certain situations and what they think it means and write it on a chart (see Tables 10.1 and 10.2). They should ask several people to check out all the possible meanings. It may take some time to find the right meanings. They may write several possibilities on the chart before they are sure of the right meaning (see Chapter 7 for more information on communication maps). They will need to work closely with the people who know and love the person to build an accurate picture of the person who is making a plan.

The best way to complete this chart is to fill in the second column first. This is the behaviour which may tell you something important about the person. They may not be consciously aware of trying to tell you something. In the first column, write down the situations when the person shows this behaviour. In the third column, write down all the possible meanings of the behaviour by asking the people who know the person well. In the fourth column, write down the best ways of supporting the person when they show this behaviour, again, asking people who know them well. It may quickly become clear what the behaviour means and what should be done to support the person or it may take a little while to get to the right answer for someone. When you think you have it right, complete a new chart which can be made available to everyone who spends time with the person.

Table 10.1 Jonathon's chart

When this is happening	Jonathon does this	We think it means	We should do this
Jonathon is reading	Sticks out his tongue	He is concentrating	Leave him alone

Table 10.2 Julie's chart

When this is happening	Julie does this	We think it means	We should do this
Sitting quietly	Bites the inside of her mouth	She is worried about something	Ask if she is OK but do not push it, if she says she is fine

People leading their plan with support

Often when professionals are describing the work they do with people with learning disabilities they talk about 'independence'. Julie, one of the authors of this chapter, trained as an occupational therapist where her work was all about helping people to be more independent. It was not long before she realised that no one is independent. We all rely on others to do things for us or with us. We all have gifts that enable us to do things for or with others. This makes us co-dependent and it is an important aspect of being part of a community where we share our lives with others as a valued citizen:

> Jean, Julie's mum, and Charles, her dad, have been married for 60 years. They have a traditional lifestyle which works for them. Jean is a great cook, which was her job before she retired. Charles has loved gardening all his life. Together they create delicious meals when all the family visit. Charles grows and prepares the vegetables and Jean makes them into tasty dishes.
>
> When Jonathon and Julie were working on a book together, Julie did the writing and Jonathon thought of most of the stories and examples that went into the book but he found writing very time-consuming. When Julie was stuck on how to phrase things in a straightforward way she asked Jonathon who used his clear thinking to provide a perfect sentence.

These are two examples of the different ways we look to others for support and share our gifts. It may be that Charles is able to do the cooking but Jean does it better. Anyway he prefers to be out in the garden. Having support to do something is not just about someone doing the things you cannot do but deciding what you like doing and sharing that out with others around us. Sometimes we can do something but we prefer others to do it for us.

Julie once supported Bill and his personal assistant to make a person centred plan. The personal assistant complained that Bill was perfectly capable of doing the housework but he always wanted those who supported him to do it for him. Bill had a 'direct payment' and paid for his support. Julie shared her own experience of employing someone to do her ironing. She was good at ironing but did not enjoy it. By paying someone to do it she was able to do her job and spend more time with her children. For Bill, someone doing his housework gave him more time to do his job selling papers and socialising with the businessmen in his community with whom he was very popular. Both Bill and Julie understood the consequences of spending money on jobs they could do for themselves but they felt it was worth it to be able to share their gifts in other parts of their lives.

It is important when planning with a person we recognise the gifts and skills that the person has so that they are not only able to demonstrate those gifts in the process of planning but that they are demonstrated in the consequences of planning.

An important aspect of supporting people to demonstrate their gifts both in planning and the consequences of planning is the decision-making agreement. This is a tool which can be used to help people to clarify what support they need to make decisions in their lives and who should help people to make those decisions, including decisions such as the ones made by Julie and Jonathon to employ someone to do some of the tasks needed to live their lives and free them up to do more pleasurable things.

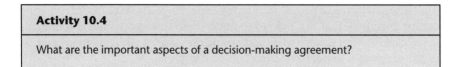

Activity 10.4

What are the important aspects of a decision-making agreement?

In order to demonstrate the important aspects of a decision-making agreement Julie and Jonathon have given examples from their lives (see Tables 10.3 and 10.4).

Table 10.3 Jonathon's decision-making agreement

Important decisions in Jonathon's life	How must I be involved?	Who makes the final decision?
Paying for my *Stargate* DVDs	Staff and Nan tell me how I can save up for them and put my money away regularly for me. They need to tell me how much I can afford	Me

Table 10.4 Julie's decision-making agreement

Important decisions in Julie's life	How must I be involved?	Who makes the final decision?
Planning a holiday with my parents and my brother's family	I need to be kept up to date about how the plans are going and when I need to send the payment for the holiday	My family decide where to go and some possible dates. I decide when it is to fit around my work

The decision-making agreement can make clear:

- when the person can make their own decisions;
- who should support them if they need help;
- who should help with which decisions;
- who may make decisions on the person's behalf;
- how they should continue to involve the person in those decisions.

People leading their own plans

Some people have strong feelings against people leading their own plans. By this they usually mean people facilitating their plans. The example of someone cutting their own hair can help us to understand that sometimes it is difficult to see clearly when you try to do something for yourself which is about you. In this situation it is better to let someone do it for you.

This does not mean that people with learning disabilities are not leading their plan. They lead by choosing:

- which type of plan is right for them;
- when they plan;
- who facilitates the plan;
- who comes to the meeting;
- where the meeting is held;
- what time the meeting is;
- deciding on the actions;
- checking the actions.

Supporting others with learning disabilities to lead their own plan

People who have experienced something for themselves often have excellent insight which cannot be matched by years of study and professional training. People with learning disabilities not only have first-hand experience if they have their own plan but they have the emotional experience of years of 'service land' which enables them to share the joys and pitfalls of planning with people. The self-advocates who have written this chapter have helped others to plan. They have facilitated plans and have given advice to others who are planning for themselves.

Training others to facilitate plans

The self-advocates writing this chapter are members of different groups who are involved in training others. To be qualified to do this they believe it is essential to have experience of developing their own plans. They use these experiences to share with others. They have also had a lot of training themselves.

Their skills, as trainers have developed with experience and they all have particular tools and techniques which they prefer to enable people to learn about planning.

Leah and Liz enjoy using role play which clearly demonstrates aspects of person centred planning. Through the role play they are able to bring humour into the training and create something which sticks in people's minds. Two of the characters in the role play Leah uses are 'Penelope Everso Posh' and 'Rachel – Voice of young people – Melarangi' where she uses the interviewing style from the *This Morning* television show to get the message across. The message of the role play being that every young person has the right to have a voice.

Jonathon is a gifted speaker. He is able to share a story with ease and confidence. He uses straightforward language which is without jargon so it is easy to understand. This is a story of his dreams which he frequently uses in training:

> *I have a dream about commanding a World War II submarine from watching war films and games. I don't think it will happen but I would like to be on a submarine. My Grandad said he would take me to Portsmouth to see the naval ships. I would love to go and see Lord Nelson's ship. I also collect models and books about military vehicles.*

In this story Jonathon demonstrates the importance of having a dream even if it might not happen and talks about some of the things that might be possible which are part of the dream.

The authors have also found it useful to share stories and experiences by having someone ask them questions which they can answer. Julie often does this in training by asking a self-advocate about themselves so that the training participants can practise working out what is *important to* and *for* people.

By training in partnership, the authors are able to use their skills and experience using a range of tools that suit the wide learning styles of their audience which include people with learning disabilities, families, friends, support staff and professionals. When anyone is learning to become a trainer, they feel nervous and lack confidence, so getting the right support to become a good trainer is essential. Liz began her training career with four questions which were read out to her, for example, what do you like about your plan? She now speaks for ten minutes and Judy who co-trains with her no longer needs to jump in and help her out. Although they both agree that they help one another out in a tricky situation and that is what good training is all about.

Leah was a shy and nervous person and when she was first asked to speak, her mum spoke on her behalf. When someone asked a question, she told her mum who would answer for her. Three weeks later she stood up in front of two hundred people and launched the White Paper in Halton. Leah says:

Now they can't shut me up. I am the voice of a young person. I used to put myself down a lot because of my Down's syndrome. I show my PATH to self-advocates. It is one of the things I am proud of. My life is a jigsaw which wouldn't be complete if someone took a piece away.

The self-advocates know that to be a good trainer they need to look back on the work they have done and think about how they can make this better. Liz has used the 'what's working/what's not working' tool to help her to think about and solve some of the problems she was having in her role as a trainer (see Table 10.5).

When creating her action plan, she needed to thinks about how to make sure that what was working continued to work as well as what could be done to change the things that were not working. When creating the action plan it is important to have the headings:

Who	Will do what	By when

Table 10.5   What's working/What's not working

	What's working	What's not working
Being a trainer	• Being paid (£20 a session) for being a trainer for the Listen To Me course/day 3 of ELP/ awareness training • Meeting new people • Training staff • Having support • More confident	• Fitting everything in! • Having an office • Rude people! • Would like a job as a trainer
Having a plan	• Sharing my plan on training and with staff who support me • Updating plan with Judy • Working with HSA	• People respecting my example plan and keeping it private • Staff ignoring what's important to me or making decisions without me
Being on Partnership Board/ meetings etc.	• Getting to know people and services and finding out information • Telling people about person centred planning and sharing my plan/PATH/community connections poster	• People speaking over me or interrupting me • Need some support in meetings • Only me to promote person centred planning • How to do a PowerPoint presentation

Sometimes people add a fourth column 'Check'. Liz was able to do most of the checking in her action plan. The action plan makes sure that everyone involved does what they are supposed to do. For Liz, it also helps her to see quickly who is doing what.

What helps people to plan for themselves?

The authors of this chapter have identified from their personal experiences some important points which help people to lead their own plans, these include circles of support, being paid, accessible plans, jargon-free language and the right to try new things.

Circles of support

People who are supporting someone to plan need to listen to the person or people who know and love them to find out who is important in their lives. A good way to do this is to draw a relationship circle. The circle will give a picture of how close the people are to the person. This is Jonathon's relationship circle (see Figure 10.2).

As the person or someone who is supporting them to plan, discovers who the important people are, then write or use graphics to record their names in the circle. The closer they are to the person, the more important they are. If they are asking other people who know and love the person, then they need to ask several people to get a full picture. For example, a day centre supporter may not know about Auntie Molly, who has known Jayne since she was a baby, who frequently visits at home and always makes Jayne laugh. Auntie Molly could easily get left out.

The person planning or those supporting them can use this information to invite people to become part of the person's circle of support. These are a group of people who agree to take on responsibilities to support the person to make sure the actions from their plan happen. They will meet up occasionally, sometimes as a whole group or part group with the person to discuss progress and sort out problems. Circles of support grow and change as the person grows and changes.

Leah has had a circle of support for a long time. In the beginning she found there were some members who were not really committed to helping her make changes in her life. Sometimes they did not turn up for meetings. Those people have now left.

She says her circle helped her to feel more confident which enabled her to speak to students at a local university in the Department of Education about inclusion. She wanted to do aromatherapy at college but the college only had a diploma course which they would not let her do. The circle helped her to think

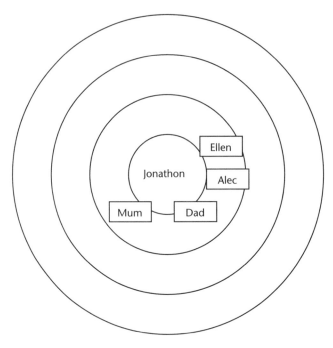

Figure 10.2   Jonathon's relationship circle.

of different ways to solve this problem. The circle also made a promise that Gemma would get involved to enable her to go out in the evening with her friends.

Being paid

Being paid for person centred planning work is important recognition of the value of that work. Many people with learning disabilities have to fight to receive payment as we saw in Liz's 'what's working/what's not working'. In the beginning she was not paid and it became an action on her PATH. She would not let it drop. In the beginning she got gift tokens. Now she is paid but no more than £20 a session or it affects her benefits. This is still an issue as it does not reflect the true worth of expert trainers.

Accessible plans

The person owns the plan so they should keep it or choose who should look after it for them. Plans must be recorded in different ways that are meaningful to the person. This can be in pictures, video tapes, symbols, etc. There may need to be more than one format to the plan. One that gives the detail that is needed for people supporting the person to know what and how they should be doing things and another that makes sense to the person. It is also important that the person gets the right support to understand the plan. Chapter 7, about 'Total Communication' describes how this should be done.

Jargon-free language

Not using long and fancy words with person centred planning that people with learning disabilities do not understand is important. If difficult words have to be used, a list of these can be recorded in the meeting so everyone understands what they mean.

The right to do new things

Recognising that people have the right to try something whether others like it or not is important. The job of people who are supporting them or the circle of support is to try and find a way for it to happen that is safe for the person.

Conclusion

People with learning difficulties are able to lead their own plans and they need good support to do this. Professionals and other people with learning disabilities have a role in giving this support. It is important that everyone involved in the planning process is able to get good training where they can learn to use the tools that have been used in this and other chapters. There needs to be good systems and practices in place to support the planning process and making sure actions happen. When all this happens people who have a learning disability will have a real chance of self determination.

Further reading

Baldwin, M. (2006) 'Person centred planning and care management with people with learning disabilities', *British Journal of Social Work*, 36: 1069–71.
Brown, H. (2000) Lecture about the 'No Secrets' research, Winchester.
Cambridge, P. and Carnaby, S. (2005) *Person Centred Planning, Care Management and People with Learning Disabilities*. London: Jessica Kingsley Publishers.
Department of Constitutional Affairs (2004) *A Guide to the Mental Capacity Bill: What Does It Mean for Me?* London: Stationery Office.
Duffy, S. (2006) *Keys to Citizenship*. Birkenhead: Paradigm.
Fulton, K. and Nicoll, T. (2006) *Hands off my plan*. Manchester: CSIP.

Kilbane, J. and Sanderson, H. (2005) 'What' and 'how': understanding professional involvement in person centred planning styles and approaches, *Learning Disability Practice*, 7(4): 16–20.

Liverpool and Manchester People First (1996) *Our Plan for Planning*. Manchester: Manchester People First.

Lunt, J. and Bassett, J. (2007) *The Best of Both Voices: Person Centred Advocacy*. Manchester: HSA Publishing. Available at: http://www.hft.org.uk/data/asset/file87.pdf

Nicoll, T. and Flood, K. (2005) 'Self advocates leading person centred planning', *Learning Disability Practice*, 8(1): 14–7.

Smull, M. and Sanderson, H. (2005) *Essential Lifestyles Planning for Everyone*. Manchester: The Learning Community – Essential Lifestyles Planning.

The Learning Community – Essential Lifestyles Planning (2001) *Listen to Me Workbook*. Manchester: The Learning Community.

11 Families leading person centred planning

Barbara Coles and Alison Short

Key issues

- Families leading planning
- Ownership urgency and action
- Family mentors
- Implementation allies
- Learning together – professionals and families
- Introducing, contributing, integrating and safeguarding

Introduction

> *The process of gathering information from other people to inform our son's plan has crystallised what we already knew about him – it has given us the confidence to take the plan forward to make changes in his life. It has given us an opportunity to regain some control over our family situation and be recognised by services as someone to work 'with' rather than 'against' in any future planning.*
>
> (A mother leading planning for her son)

A complete mix of family members from parents, siblings, grandparents and aunts have become involved in the work of families leading planning and in many instances the result has been that their relative has achieved real power in shaping the course of their life. The input from these families has also highlighted the qualities and skills they naturally have. This has led to flexible and responsive supports based on the person's plan. As a further outcome the work has increased the number of families who are telling positive stories about how they were supported to learn to plan by other family members and the welcoming response they received from some services.

Our work is pushing the boundaries of professional thinking by challenging the common assumption that families stifle their family member by placing an emphasis on care and protection rather than encouraging autonomy, and the belief that, as a consequence, families are not in the best position to take the lead in planning. Although this issue is complex, in our experience, these two elements are not mutually exclusive and in most instances families get the balance right!

Some, but not enough, professionals are championing the shift in practice set out above and understand that they need to work differently when implementing a person centred plan that has been facilitated by a family member. This chapter discusses how families can take the lead in person centred planning and how professionals can help support them with this initiative. It describes the work that families have been doing in recent years to enable this to happen, as well as some of the outcomes of this work. In addition, we introduce the concept of 'Implementation allies', these being helpful professionals who support family members who are taking the lead in planning. This chapter also describes the training and support family members have received and the 'practical next steps' which professionals need to take in order to enhance the work done by families. Indeed, we argue that professionals can only be successful in their role if they establish a good working relationship with family members who have chosen to take the lead in planning. Only then will they ensure that an individual is provided with support and resources to match her or his own goals and support requirements, rather than them having to fit into the predetermined plans of professionals and service systems.

Indeed, family involvement in, or leadership of, planning in this way has multiple benefits: for the individual, their families (their voices are listened to and respected) and professionals (in terms of the planning done by service workers, for example, transition plans, core assessments, etc.).

Authors' relationship explained

We feel that it would be helpful to the reader to set out our entwined journey as we come from very different starting points. Our stories offer a clear example of how strong working relationships can grow between family members and professionals if both parties are prepared to learn through constantly listening to each other and acting on what they are hearing. In terms of our relationship, we have been performing a dance whereby sometimes we made up our own steps and danced independently of each other and at other times danced in unison. The analogy of dance is expanded on in the summary of this chapter.

Barbara set up Families Leading Planning UK, which provides learning, training and development opportunities for family members. She is actively involved in supporting her son to be able to live a lifestyle of his choosing by directly managing his support and living arrangements. Alison, on the other hand, trained as an Occupational Therapist but now works as a consultant and trainer. The authors first got to know each other when Alison was the manager of a local respite service. In a time of crisis and need in Barbara's family's life, Alison was part of a team of people who could not offer Barbara and her family a service that was desperately needed. This was based on the assumption that their son was too difficult to support – a premise that is not generally conducive to a good working relationship!

However, in recent years Barbara and Alison have been learning together and supporting families, demonstrating how people working in services and family members can forge strong working relationships. For Alison, the key point that unlocked the potential from a 'professional perspective' providing services for people like Barbara's son was when she stopped working within the boundaries of the 'labels' that had been placed upon him. By taking a person centred approach, she started to get to know him as an individual human being. Had this happened at the point of the initial request for support, Alison believes there would have been a very different outcome for the family.

The authors believe that their working relationship developed because they each took off their 'blinkers' and really got to know each other on a personal level – a trip that brought together a group of 'professionals' and family members canoeing in America (in the dark and lit only by their headlights) was a definitive turning point in their relationship. Alison became extremely scared of the precarious situation she found herself in and needed physical help to get back to shore. Barbara's (who offered this support) reflection of this experience shows that until this point she had only ever seen Alison in her professional role – this incident 'humanised' her – 'the shoe was on the other foot' as she was now the one in desperate need of support! This is an example of what families have to offer 'professionals' and other people who work in services. Families are particularly good in terms of creativity, compassion and developing shared insights for action. We have since on many occasions, been witness to this type of 'relationship transformation' between family members and professionals.

The contribution of families and their role in person centred planning

Person centred thinking and planning is a central theme of most current policy guidance where the emphasis is clearly on the individual and their families being in control of the direction of their support. It is therefore vital for professionals to be able to see how families bring their experience to bear within this process and to have the opportunities to develop their own skills in light of this change.

Person centred planning (Department of Health 2001b: 12) *'is a process of continual listening and learning focusing on what is important to someone now and for the future: and acting on this in alliance with their family and friends'*. It naturally places people who have learning disabilities in the context of their family and community. People recognise that families want their opinions and expertise about their relatives to be an integral part of decision-making about the people they love. This is poignant, as over half of the people who have learning disabilities in England live with their families, and yet the learning and implementation of person centred planning to date have been predominantly within the service system. Dowson (1991: 12) describes an absurdity in human services whereby *'activities which ordinary people undertake casually, for their own sake, and which might provide people with learning difficulties with the same kind of opportunities, are defined as therapies or schemes. This ensures that the people who do them are still firmly within the service arena.'* Furthermore, Mount (1994: 103) warns *'when the system takes over the "futures planning process", the activity immediately loses its power, flexibility and responsiveness, quickly becoming one more intrusive, insensitive and ineffective activity'*.

Rudkin and Rowe (2001) argued that this happened during the initial implementation of person centred planning. They found a 70 per cent non-adherence to a person centred plan six months after the plan had been implemented and we conclude from this that person centred planning is subverted by the service system. Robertson et al. (2005) found that person centred planning is more likely to be implemented if the person lives near their family. In short, working alongside families that are either leading the planning process, or being supported to plan is going to be an increasing feature of practice in the future:

> *When we are involved, our families plans tend to be more sustainable and outcomes ongoing because whatever happens we families will always be there, we know the person well because we really listen to them and we get others to listen to them through ongoing collective learning.*
>
> (A mother supporting other families to plan)

The guidance *Person Centred Approaches* (Department of Health 2001b) recommends that local authorities invest in finding ways for families to take the lead in planning and be full and active partners in this process should they wish.

Activity 11.1

- Are families in your area able to lead on plans for their loved one if they wish?
- What is done to help them achieve this?
- What difficulties do they experience in doing this?

Dumas et al. (2002) found that families in the USA could be self-efficacious in person centred planning but identified key factors that limited them, such as the low expectations of families about their ability to affect the process or outcomes of planning. The evidence that we are finding is that even though families are very able to develop the skills to affect change in the lives of the people they love by using person centred planning approaches, they are often held back by the distinctly traditional beliefs and practices of professionals: *'How can families possibly plan? They don't have access to photocopiers!'* This is Alison's reflection on her early experiences of supporting families with person centred planning. She recalls how her view had been so clouded by her own model of professional practice. Alison had totally missed the point as planning within Alison's world had been a very process- and 'paper-driven' exercise, hence the link to the photocopier. She soon realised that family members were able to produce plans that incorporated the richest of information. And what's more, the plans were generally completed quickly and effectively. She also heard about how using the local photocopier at the corner shop had opened up a possibility of friendship for the person whose plan was being developed!

Families come to the process of person centred planning for a variety of reasons

There are always going to be family members who start their journey of learning by wanting to develop a plan and then use it as a weapon to batter services with but, on the whole, families are coming to the planning process with an absolute need to find a way forward for the people they love. Often this is because the service system has failed to provide it, as in Barbara's case. Family members do want to be able to work successfully with professionals and have a process whereby their expertise around the person they love and support can be recognised. More often than not, however, the relationships family members have with professionals have totally broken down. The planning process enables the relationships to be reformed in a proactive and positive manner that recognises everyone's contributions. In most cases, the family member has initiated the process themselves.

Ownership, urgency and action

Family members bring immense assets to the planning process, for example, 'ownership', 'urgency' and 'action' (Provencal 1987). *Ownership* refers to people having the power and control over their lives and being the key to their own solutions. *Urgency* is about human services understanding that the pace of the calendar and time moves the same for people who have impairments as those who do not. Families are acutely aware of this flow of time. Focusing on *action* is also critical in order to address and move on with solutions and ensuring that life moves on at the same pace as anybody else. As 'content' and 'process' experts (see below), families often have the key to the solutions for the situations that they are trying to address. Family ownership of these solutions is vital if people's lives are not to be over-professionalised. It should be no surprise that families are able to facilitate quality plans which lead to positive action and outcomes as families are much more aware of the pace at which time moves on for the person they love and the urgent need to address the issues that affect them. For example, Ann (a mum who has recently been learning about person centred thinking and planning and who has also facilitated a plan for Alfie, one of her sons) clearly demonstrates the concept of 'ownership', 'urgency' and 'action'.

Ann became involved in person centred planning because she needed to find some method of sorting out the thoughts in her head about Alfie. Ann knew that Alfie and her family were not being able to access the resources he and her family required. She felt that professionals were not listening to her or taking her seriously. With support Ann facilitated an Essential Lifestyle Plan with and for Alfie. She took Alfie's plan with her when she and Alfie went to their next appointment at Great Ormond Street Hospital for his neurological assessment:

> *I explained that I wanted them to be able to see the detail of Alfie's life and read other people's observations of him as well as mine and my husband's. While Alfie was completing a range of tests, the different members of the team took time to read Alfie's plan. Finally, after years and years of neuro and psychological assessments, Alfie was given a diagnosis of Asperger's Syndrome. This was the first time I wasn't treated like a neurotic, hysterical parent!*

Ann added:

> *I want to thank you for all the help you have given me in developing the plan so far and acknowledge what a powerful tool it has been in supporting Alfie and the rest of our family.*

Ann's story of 'ownership', 'urgency' and 'action' continues as she is supported by other families taking the lead in planning at her second son, Joseph's person centred transition meeting which she initiated. This is what Joseph's Dad and Ann said about the meeting:

> *I feel the meeting was both informative and helpful. My mind has been set at rest and I can see Joseph not having any problems with his transition to secondary school. The professionals actually seemed human! I am now confident about Joseph's future at his new school.*
>
> (Joseph's Dad)

> *Really loved it. So different from all the other review meetings which we have been to every year since Joseph was 3. It's the first time Joseph has come to a meeting and been able to stay for the whole thing. The first time that he was really being listened to. The first time I didn't feel like an intruder or an annoyance. I felt validated and listened to. It has given me real hope for his future – if everyone's actions are kept to and using person centred principles throughout his time at school, things will really change for the better.*
>
> (Ann, Joseph's Mum)

Ann is using the information gathered at Joseph's meeting to inform Joseph's Essential Lifestyle Plan. Ann's story of 'ownership', 'urgency' and 'action', however, does not stop here:

> *I wanted to let you know how powerful the person centred review questions have been for us again. I had to attend a review for my youngest son, this week. He doesn't have any learning difficulties just an expressive speech and language disorder called severe phonological disorder. I used the person centred review questions you sent to me in preparation for Joseph's meeting as a basis to informally find out what I needed to know about his school experiences and support needs. During the meeting I asked each person what they liked and admired about him and heard some amazing things, some of which even I didn't know about him. However, the most surprising response was how emotional other people got. The Special Educational Needs Co-ordinator (SENCO) said that it was the first time she had heard such positive and personal statements about a child at a review and she even had tears in her eyes! It really makes all types of reviews a totally different experience for everybody concerned. I was also able to come home and tell my son some of the really nice things that people had said about him.*

The above extracts highlight how, through using person centred thinking and planning skills and tools, families – as people not employed by services – are able to apply positive pressure for change outside the system. Professionals are not always able to take on this role. They can act as 'Allies' (see below) but there are things that need to come directly from people who receive support. With this in mind, local areas need to think about the following questions: *Who is controlling person centred thinking and planning?*, *Who holds the technical expertise?* and *Who is doing the learning?* Effective planning requires attention to change *within* and *beyond* the service system.

It is also worth remembering that families are 'there for the long haul' and act as a critical 'safeguard' to quality as service workers come and go, therefore this type of investment in families in terms of supporting them to learn about and take the lead on person centred planning is long overdue. In addition, families can take on the role of 'critical friend' for professionals, in taking on this role they can 'drive up' the quality of professional practice. Indeed, many professionals reading this chapter will recall that the best lectures they went to when training were those where people with disabilities or their families led the sessions. In our experience family members who are learning about planning are more than willing to help professionals with their training by sharing personal experiences and stories. This enriches the learning of professionals as it enables them to see their intervention in the context of people's lives. Having family members leading the planning process and families and professionals learning about and planning together gives a heightened purpose to service development/provision and community development that is sustainable.

Roles within the planning process

Smull and Sanderson (2005) look at two specific roles within the planning process – that of 'content experts' and 'process experts'. 'Content experts' know what a plan should say as they are the experts in their own lives or the lives of the people they love, whereas 'process experts' know how to help someone through the planning process to get an outcome.

Activity 11.2

- What approaches can you use to help you avoid being the content expert when working with a family?
- How do you feel as a professional when a family takes on this role?

We have often found the role of the professional has been ascribed as the process expert and in some cases professional practice has also taken over the 'content' of people's plans. When families take the lead, we are redefining these roles as the family member can also become the process expert. In our experience of supporting family members to learn, families have clearly demonstrated their competence in using the person centred thinking tool 'what's working/what's not working' from different perspectives:

> *Planning made me stop and think about what my son wants – not just what me or his Dad want for him.*

> *I've learnt so much about my daughter through planning in this way. I need now to question myself as to why I do what I do in the way that I do it. I need to change not my daughter.*

> *I was able to write a detailed plan for my daughter with the support of my peers.*

In terms of best practice therefore, professionals in their role of *safeguarding* person centred approaches should be actively looking at how they can support 'content experts' in becoming 'process experts' should they wish. Families Leading Planning UK is just one initiative that is addressing this through structured learning and development designed with families and for families.

How families are learning to take the lead in person centred planning

Figure 11.1 shows a description of the focused effort called 'Families Leading Planning'. It shows how learning is structured and how professionals can support this structure.

The following are quotations from family members expressing how learning in this way helped some of them to see their family member differently and others to have their understanding of their loved ones affirmed:

> *I am enjoying the challenge of starting an Essential Lifestyle Plan and getting to know my daughter better.*

> *Even though my plan is not yet complete, I am confident enough to start the ball rolling for direct payments. I wouldn't have done it without the knowledge and confidence this course has given me.*

> *I feel clearer and more focused for the future.*

> *I never thought other people would know my son so well.*

> *Through planning I have learnt to love my son again and I'm so proud he is mine – all I used to hear were all the negative comments about his behaviour!*

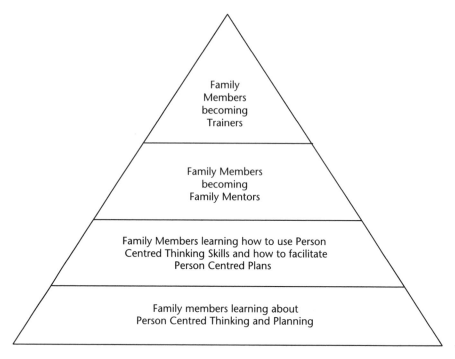

Figure 11.1   The structure of Families Leading Planning

I'm so pleased that I did the plan and that my son has got something he did not have before. I know him so much better.

Working together with other family members and sharing our concerns, positive stories, obstacles and helping each other has been so helpful to me.

I have learnt how to step out of the box of being 'Mum' and look at her as an individual.

Families Leading Planning UK's 'Essential Lifestyle Planning' Course

Wherever possible, the individual themselves should develop their own plan (see Chapter 10 for more information on this) but where this is not possible and they need support to do this, then family and friends are ideally placed to develop a plan with and for them. Families leading planning courses are being delivered in a number of areas. Typically these follow the format outlined in Box 11.1.

Box 11.1 Families leading planning courses

Important considerations

- Course members will be adult learners
- Interactive approaches to learning are preferable
- Support systems need to be in place for support during and after the course
- Family mentorship and leadership programmes are important infrastructures
- Skills in quality monitoring are crucial

Structure of the course

- Design Day – this makes sure that the course is tailored to the local context
- Awareness Day introducing Person Centred Thinking and Planning
- Gathering information from What You Know
- Gathering information from Others and Health Action Planning
- Two days for developing the plan
- Action Planning
- Implementation
- Ongoing learning and local development

Course evaluation

- use the 4 plus 1 person centred planning questions
  - What have we tried?
  - What have we learnt?
  - What are we pleased about?
  - What are we concerned about?
  - Based on what we know now, what are our next steps?

More information is available from www.familiesleadingplanning.co.uk

---

Family members are now also reporting how they are able to use the person centred thinking skills in transferable ways in other aspects of their lives. Family members have said that this has given them greater personal confidence. This is also relevant to the skills people develop in being family trainers and family mentors.

Family trainers

Family trainers lead the course. This is paramount as the following quotation from an older family member suggests:

You know what we are talking about just hearing what you have been doing to support your son and the struggles and barriers that you encountered means that we will listen to you whereas you (addressing a non-family trainer) *although you are kind and supportive and say all the right things, it's not the same, you don't really know what it is like for us and anyway I expect you will be moving to a new job soon and we'll never see you again . . . whereas she will be around for as long as her son needs her.*

The training that family trainers receive has emerged from our work in the UK. This included learning from family members who informally developed person centred plans, and also from those who engaged in structured learning on a course in 2001. This course was developed collectively with family members and Helen Sanderson Associates. Family trainers continue to act as family mentors to other family members interested in working in this field. Additionally, we are now at the stage where families are asking for professionals whom they trust to have the opportunity to co-train and be accredited for their skills alongside family members. This again fosters great partnership working.

Family mentors

A family mentor is someone who has been supported to learn how to facilitate a person centred plan with and for their own family member and has an interest in supporting other families who wish to do the same. Family mentors may find themselves working in a variety of settings, which requires many skills. Training as a family mentor on an Essential Lifestyle Planning Course provides the trainee with the key foundation skills necessary to ensure quality planning and implementation – in an environment where she or he is able to access individual learning and support tailored to meet their needs. This is also enhanced by group discussions and problem solving, a process that stands them in good stead should they wish to work as a lone facilitator in the future.

The role of a family mentor is to help other families to learn and understand about person centred thinking and planning and help with the implementation of plans facilitated in this way. They connect with, listen to, support and encourage the family they are working with. Although the amount of support they provide is likely to be different for each family, it should consist of as much assistance as is required, but no more than is needed or wanted. Many family mentors also act as 'system navigators' to those they are supporting, as they are likely to know the context of 'how things are done locally' just as 'professional allies' should.

The development of allies

Initially our efforts focused on family members learning about person centred thinking and planning. The experience of the family below shows that this is just one piece of the jigsaw:

> *I have experienced first hand the progress that my son has been able to achieve through using person centred planning but have struggled in the maintenance of this because of the lack of guidance, understanding and external support. I have had to rely on the 'goodwill' input of 'experts' to whom I was eternally grateful, but ultimately the continuity has been left to ourselves as a family, which can sometimes be counter-productive if there are not enough outside influences to make changes happen and to enable us to effectively problem solve.*

It became clear very quickly that there needed to be opportunities for local workers to learn alongside families and to have an understanding of how to respond and support these particular families when implementing their plans. In light of the above quotation, we asked ourselves the question 'Do professionals need to respond differently to the families?' The answer, of course, was 'Yes'. So we began supporting professionals to develop skills for the role of 'allies'. It was not enough, though, to assume that professional training would have prepared workers to support a family member when they have chosen to lead the planning process and help with the implementation of their family member's plan. So far, allies have come from many professional backgrounds, including care management, social work, and community nursing.

What do allies do?

Allies support a family member to implement the person centred plans that they have facilitated. Stone (1999) said:

> *An ally means getting alongside people and working with them to make sure that any changes have the best possible impact on the person . . . An ally understands how the system works and tries to use what is good in the system.*

Activity 11.3
How could you act as an ally to support families who are trying to plan in your area?

Acting as an ally to families means using professional skills, but in a different way. Allies need to be able to work across boundaries and support families from a different starting position. Allies with professional backgrounds must be able to give support, yet not lead families into planning with service solutions in mind, and not inadvertently take over the planning process.

The competency of families who are learning about planning should be respected at all times. The lure of the 'helping professional' may be towards a 'quick fix' and in the current balance of power families may well feel that they have to listen to the professional and act in accordance with them. In this event, the potency of the planning process may well be lost. In times of crisis, services tend to resort to 'quick fixes' but these reduce the number of possible options for people.

Professionals acting as allies supporting families on a recent course began to see things from a different perspective. They started to value the amount of hands-on support families provide. They also noted how family members, whom they had been supporting prior to this course, responded differently to them in this context. The following are what this particular group of professionals/allies learned:

- Families are more knowledgeable of what is available and are not settling for traditional services.
- Families are breaking down communication barriers.
- Families seem more confident in questioning services.
- Families are challenging 'bad practice'.
- Families have valuable information that needs to be shared.
- Service providers have learned more about individuals and the need for consistency.
- Shifting control from services to individuals and families is very positive.
- It is challenging us to find new services and to be flexible in our thinking.
- Our hope is that more families can be supported to do their own planning.
- Families will become mentors and trainers to other families and this will lead to services becoming more responsive.
- The culture will change away from 'we know best' to become a shared view.

These allies said that there were specific requirements of an ally in order to be able to make a difference in supporting families to take the lead in planning:

- clarity of roles outside the course in terms of supporting implementation of plans;

- clear concise commitment to undertake this role;
- commitment from senior managers along with an undertaking to release staff and skilled facilitators to provide support when and where it is needed;
- negotiation of time required;
- clear value-based principles need to be demonstrated;
- good listening and hearing skills are required;
- a non-judgemental attitude;
- a clear commitment to equality and diversity;
- that the person turns up when they have said they will.

One ally who has direct experience of supporting families to take the lead in planning in this way said: *'This has been a powerful experience that has changed the way I think, view situations, and work with families.'*

Person centred planning co-ordinators can also act as an ally. As such, their involvement in any work in this area is important, particularly where they can act as a link between families and the local Partnership Board. Likewise the support of local person centred planning facilitators acting as 'allies' or 'thinking partners' can be a great local resource. It is important to remember that people taking this role, whatever their background, must be briefed in advance about the purpose of their participation.

In spite of the initiatives we have described, there are still those professionals whose attitudes can hinder the process of person centred planning led by families. In doing this they often risk duplication of efforts when scarce resources prevail. For example, one professional learning to be an ally said that they thought their role was to agree and sign off the person centred plan the family had facilitated. This logic is often used by services showing their need to control and agree plans within resource constraints and protecting their profession. The role of the ally is in fact to support the process, not to sign it off or assure its quality. However, should a person centred plan become the support plan in the context of self-directed support, then the plan will need to be signed off by a representative of the Local Authority (see Chapter 12). This is, however, a very different concept to that of the unnecessary process of signing off a person centred plan.

Activity 11.4

Why do some professionals find it difficult to support people when they are planning and act as allies?

Another professional exploring her role in relation to families taking the lead in planning said that she would not trust a plan that had been written by a family member and would have to get to know the person herself. She said it was her professional duty and need. This was an interesting insight into the mind of this particular professional as she was not able to see that the voice of the individual coming through the plan was the same voice, whether it was facilitated by a family member or a professional facilitator. Indeed, by feeling she had to get to know the person, she would have been using scarce professional time – time that would have been better spent helping the family member to get answers to their questions, and ensuring that decisions generated from the planning meetings were implemented.

We have, nevertheless, found that professionals are able to change their working practices with families using person centred thinking approaches. Moreover, they have welcomed the opportunity of working in this way. The training that we have provided for allies has focused on:

- exploring ways in which professionals and others can best support families in this initiative;
- identifying what constitutes helpful or unhelpful support in this context;
- identifying what resources and attributes professionals and others can bring to bear in working in this way with families;
- clarifying, understanding and developing the role as an ally;
- enabling professionals and others to directly problem solve issues that may arise when helping families with this process;
- helping professionals and others to be clear about how their practice can develop in ways that enable families who are planning to be supported effectively.

We have found that it has been beneficial for families and allies to learn about 'action planning' and 'ongoing learning' jointly. Families have consistently said that they wish to lead the development of the plan, but really want to be 'mum' or 'dad', etc. at the action-planning meeting. For this reason they welcomed someone familiar to them facilitating the process at that stage.

Professionals have told us that they want to be able to practise and support families in this way by having that 'human connection' – by 'breaking the rules' and 'thinking outside the box' and generally having more personal commitment and time, seeing things through, daring to be different, having good information, exploring things with people, stretching people's vision, encouraging, standing back and personal reflection. Working in partnership helps this to happen.

In light of the above therefore, just what *has* worked and what *has not* been helpful to families in their role of leading planning? In Box 11.2 we summarise some of the issues that have emerged so far.

Box 11.2 What's working/what's not working

What's working

- It is happening – professionals are working alongside families.
- Families feel that their knowledge is being recognised by professionals.
- Some professionals are using the plans facilitated by family members to inform assessment and care plans.
- Families feel the difference in this way of working.
- Changes can be seen in the lives of individuals.
- Energy and enthusiasm are flowing in both directions.
- There is a genuine willingness by professionals to support families in this way because it has helped them in their own roles.
- Professionals are being trained by family members to support families and co-train with them.

What's not working

- Despite extensive guidance and training about person centred planning, some professionals are still giving families incorrect information about planning.
- Local authorities are only concentrating on building staff/organisational capacity rather than supporting family development in this area of training.
- A care manager saying, 'Well, these plans are not recognised around here.'
- Families reporting that plans are being ignored.
- Families saying that they are viewed with suspicion by professionals because they have led the planning process.
- Families saying that workers have to come into people's homes to assess them and do not use the plan as a starting point to gather information about the person. They ask the question, 'If the plan speaks for the person, why do professionals feel that they have to get so involved or "double check" it in some way?'

Working together: what professionals need to know and do to support families that are taking/have taken the lead in person centred planning

The ways in which professionals are able to engage in person centred planning was articulated in the model proposed by Kilbane and Sanderson (2004). This model identified four different ways in which professionals could contribute to person centred planning. These are: 'introducing', 'contributing', 'safe-guarding' and 'implementing' (see Figure 11.2).

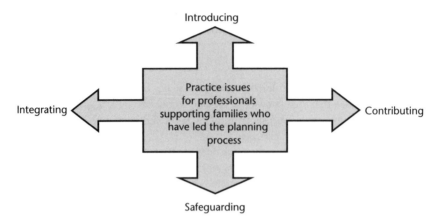

Figure 11.2   The person centred planning model for professionals
Source: Adapted from Kilbane and Sanderson (2005)

Introducing families to person centred planning

Professionals are in a position of power in terms of 'doing' person centred planning as this is where investment in training and development is predominately placed. Families who have led plans have been in the minority as a result of this. This is not because they do not wish to lead plans. Rather, it is because they have not always been given the opportunity, even though the Best Practice Guidance clearly calls for family members to be informed about person centred planning as well as resources and materials to be made available to those families who wish to take the lead in planning for their loved ones.

Activity 11.5

How could you support families to begin to plan with their loved ones?

Here are examples of ways in which to get started:

- Professionals leading person centred planning locally need to map out where local family groups are and develop a strategy for sharing information with them, if this has not already been done.
- Professionals should work together with local family leadership initiatives to co-design development in this area.
- The training opportunities that are available to professionals should be opened up to include family members, as this makes the experience of the training so much richer, and lays the foundations for building good working relationships.

- Professionals should encourage and support family members with experience of person centred planning by giving them opportunities to talk to other families and carers, informing them of what person centred planning *is* and *is not*, and what opportunities are available locally for them to get involved if they so wish.
- The community team should be used as a resource point for this initial information giving. Setting up a resource library that is accessible to families at convenient times is helpful. This resource should have information on person centred thinking and planning specifically for families.
- Professionals should use person centred thinking tools as determined in the person centred thinking model in Box 11.3 to aid their introduction to families and to negotiate their roles. This is a way of gradually introducing the approach in practice and in conversations with families. (Families who have developed plans will find it helpful to be supported in such a coherent manner.)

For example, using the tool 'Important to and for' will enable the professional to negotiate accurately how best to support a family. Using this tool can be the starting point for positive communications and for building trust, as it does not leave things to chance. It also allows the professional to track their relationship with the family as both parties learn about working together in a positive manner. It is also an excellent tool to show evidence of reflective practice (see Box 11.3).

In addition, 'The doughnut' model (see Chapter 3) (Core responsibilities; Judgement and creativity; Not our responsibility) can be used to decide collectively with families who is going to do what. The examples in Table 11.1 show how this can have regard for your professional role while at the same time connecting with the family's priorities and expectations. It is important that professionals know where a family is happy for them to use their judgement and creativity and what is exclusively the role of the family.

Contributing and integrating person centred planning led by families into your practice

'Contributing' and 'integrating' into practice person centred planning led by families are paramount. The contribution of professionals in supporting this process over time will, inevitably, lead to learning new ways of integrating these two elements into professional procedures and practice methods, for example:

- using information from plans to influence professional practice (for example, arranging meetings or activities with the person in the

---

Box 11.3 Person centred thinking introduction model

What is important to the family:

- That things are explicated clearly.
- Do not make assumptions that we know about things – check this out by asking us.
- That we can be cross.
- That people do not assume that they know what is right for my son and me and my family.
- That I can be contacted any time on my mobile.
- That we as a family like to have fun and want our relationship to go with a swing, but we expect people to be serious when they need to be.

What you need to know or do as professionals:

- Make sure you do not use jargon or 'service speak'.
- Ask us about what we know and understand about a specific topic.
- When we are cross, it will not always be with you, take the time to find out what is going on and help to put things right if you can.
- Make sure you have my mobile number.
- Make sure you are flexible as this works best for us.
- Do not worry if you get stuck – just be honest and tell us so we can work it out together.

What we are learning together:

Table 11.1   The doughnut model

	Core responsibility	Judgement and creativity	Not our paid responsibility
My job role	To develop a Health Action Plan with and for your son	How I can collect the information and how the information is recorded	I can only provide advice and guidance on how this is to be used to those supporting your son
What works for you and your son?	Having a pictorial version of this Using what information already exists in my son's plan to inform the Health Action Plan That you identify health actions in line with what is important to my son	How you look for information that will help us to answer the questions we have raised in the plan regarding my son's health	We would not want you going to my son's GP to ask questions – we can do that as we have a good relationship with her

    mornings if their plan indicates that this is a good time for them; using learning logs as tools to gather further information);

- recording outcomes, new learning and actions resulting from professional interventions into someone's person centred plan.

Finding ways of doing this together will become easier if a shared knowledge of the person centred thinking tools has provided a common language. The role of professionals as allies and as contributors to a person centred plan is essential if these plans are to be implemented.

We already know that there is a greater likelihood of change happening in people's lives when the plan is developed in partnership. When a family member is taking the lead, professionals could be asked to contribute to the plan at the 'information gathering stage'. This helps with all aspects of the planning process – the plan's development, its 'actioning' and contributing to the ongoing learning.

However, in order to contribute, a professional must be invited to do so by the family member facilitating the plan. This implies that professionals must understand the proper focus of their contribution, and be committed to completing any resulting actions. In essence, professionals must appreciate that they are engaged in 'sharing power', not having power alone.

Thinking about how professional reports and assessments can be structured differently offers practical ways forward in terms of 'contributing' to planning with families. One example of this is provided by a young professional who was running a summer scheme for children who have learning disabilities. This professional was aware that families in a locality were learning how to take the lead in planning. Each year, part of her role was to write up a report about each child on the scheme. This year she wrote the reports under the headings of a plan so that the families were able to transfer this information quickly and easily into their child's plan. She wrote about what they 'liked and admired' about the children from their time spent together, as well as what she had found out about what was 'important to and for' the young person during activities.

It is equally important that professionals should recognise the negative impact they have on families when they do *not* support the planning process families are engaged in. Such unsupportive attitudes have had a devastating effect on families who have invested time in plan development. Working actively together will make good use of professionals' and families' time and resources. Below is an account of how a care manager for transition was able to use a plan that had been led by a family member to its full potential:

> *Invariably Community Care Assessments aim to reflect exactly this sort of information (vulnerabilities, interests, level of independence, etc.) and care managers, being restricted in the amount of time they can spend getting*

> *to know the person, often need to involve members of family, staff, etc. to complete assessments. However, as with Rob's case, person centred planning can help a great deal in the assessment process, ensuring the needs and wishes of the individual are fully expressed. Perhaps without the person centred plan, as Rob's care manager, I may not have been able to present as strong a case to the Learning Disability Team, because I wouldn't have fully understood his needs and vulnerabilities myself.*

The contribution of professionals to plans that are being facilitated by families can improve the working relationship necessary for implementation, but, more importantly, it shows that people care:

> *The meeting was great – I had only expected a few staff but the whole staff team came to meet with me – it was lovely. It reinforced what I thought but I learnt lots more about my son – really learnt how much paid support staff know and care about him – fantastic.*

Professionals also need to recognise that not all families will want to lead plans. Families should not to be judged as a result. Under these circumstances the responsibility of professionals, when the family requests support in the planning process, is to provide a link to a facilitator. The Best Practice Guidance calls for the development of a pool of resources to be able to support families in this way. There should also be an agreed local process for developing family mentors and trainers to support other families to lead planning.

Safeguarding person centred planning

Families have a significant role to play in respect of safeguarding the quality of training in person centred thinking and planning as well as in quality-reviewing plans as it is the people whom they love who are directly affected by poor quality planning.

Families have been contributing to the internal quality reviewing of plans through 'peer review'; that is an integral part of the Families Leading Planning initiative. It is recommended that Person Centred Planning Co-ordinators, family trainers/mentors support the development of 'communities of practice' where families and professionals get together to learn from each other on a regular basis.

It is vitally important too that more people other than professionals are involved in safeguarding the quality of plans and planning processes (we all know that having more people involved in someone's life acts as a powerful safeguard against the abuse of vulnerable people). We can set this in the context of the Best Practice Guidance for Partnership Boards: 'Families Leading Person Centred Planning: How are we doing? Where are we going?' http://www.valuingpeople.gov.uk/PCPGuidance.htm commissioned by *Valuing People* (Department of Health 2004). In this Guidance, Partnership Boards are expected to enable families to take the lead in planning if they wish to do so. These key questions were set out to enable local areas to measure how well they were doing in supporting this initiative:

1   Are families informed about person centred planning?
2   Do families have the opportunity to learn about how to lead person centred planning?
3   Are families who do not want to or feel they cannot lead the plan given support?
4   Are families who lead the planning process given ongoing support?
5   Are families influencing the local development and quality of person centred planning for Partnership Boards, for example, is person centred planning changing people's lives for the better?
6   Are families leading planning linked to *Valuing People's* priority groups?

Unfortunately, however, the situation is that even after six years, planning that is truly person centred and owned by the person and their family remains the province of special initiatives and exceptional good practice.

Conclusion

Picking up on the analogy of 'dance' as mentioned earlier on in the chapter in terms of our relationship (the authors), Dowson (1991) uses the same analogy to contrast the operation of the service system with the style of informal family and community life. Community life is represented as a dance, which celebrates individuality:

> *Someone may offer a rhythm and a chant to start with, but each dancer takes them up and varies them according to her own inclinations. Consequently there is no guarantee that there will be any coherence between the dancers though interestingly, most of the time a complex and dynamic pattern is present. There are no given steps or fixed sequences: the dancers do not work out in advance what movements they will make but trust their bodies to express the swirling rhythm and spirit of the dance. Sometimes when one of the dancers feels inclined, she may move to the centre of the group and dance on her own. The others watch, delighting in the way her spontaneous movements celebrate the person that she is.*

In contrast, the service system follows a dance which strives to achieve coherence and unity at the expense of individuality, and where:

> *The rhythm, tune, and the movements have already been established – the aim is to perform what somebody else has devised. The rhythm is definite and unchanging, enabling the dancers to move together. The dancers are trying to achieve perfection: absolute unity, total adherence to the given steps, always to the beat. The less individual they appear, the better. Occasionally – at pre-determined points – one dancer might perform alone. The other dancers look on while he demonstrates his athleticism and skill.*
>
> (Dowson 1991)

It is no wonder therefore, that families and professionals sometimes find it hard to 'get with the beat' when they are dancing in such different ways. Each dance has focus and energy in helping change to happen for people. But the established rhythms or freedom of movement can get in the way of co-operation. What we have experienced in our work with families is that person centred thinking and planning offers both families and professionals a chance to choreograph a new dance. As there are no pre-determined steps to learn, they can dance together making new steps and rhythms. This dance is starting to show where family members have been given the opportunity to have an active part to play in the planning process, the outcome has been instrumental in bringing about significant change in the lives of the people they love and support who are, of course, the very focus of this collective dance!

Annotated bibliography

Families Leading Planning Pack, www.elpnet.net
This pack has been developed through our shared learning as part of the Essential Lifestyle Planning Learning Community. It has been specifically designed for family members to learn about a particular type of person centred planning called 'Essential Lifestyle Planning'. Throughout the material you will find comments that have been made by families as they have undertaken the planning process.

This learning aid helps families develop a plan which will enable them to discover and describe:

- what is important to their family member now and for the future;
- what support their family member wants and needs to keep them healthy and safe.

Once a plan has been developed, the pack describes how it can be put into practice and how to capture new learning about the person as our understanding of them deepens over time.

References

Department of Health (2001a) *Valuing People: A New Strategy for Learning Disability for the 21st Century*. London: Department of Health.

Department of Health (2001b) *Person Centred Approaches: Planning with People. Guidance for Implementation Groups*. London: HMSO.

Department of Health (2004) *Person Centred Approaches: Next Steps Families Leading Person Centred Planning: How Are We Doing? Where Are We Going? Good Practice Ideas for Partnership Boards*. London: The Stationery Office.

Dowson, S. (1991) *Moving to the Dance or Service Culture and Community Care*. London: Values Into Action.

Dumas, S., De La Garza, D., Seay, P. and Becker, H. (2002) ' "I don't know how they made it happen, but they did": efficacy perceptions in using a person centred planning process', in S. Holburn and P. Vietze (eds) *Research into Person Centred Planning*. Boston, MA: Paul H. Brookes Publishing Co.

Kilbane, J. and Sanderson, H. (2004) 'What' and 'how': understanding professional involvement in person centred planning styles and approaches', *Journal of Learning Disabilities*, 7(4): 16–20.

Mount, B. (1994) 'Benefits and limitations of personal futures planning', in V. Bradley, J. Ashbaugh and B. Blaney (eds), *Creating Individual Supports for People with Developmental Disabilities*. Baltimore, MD: Paul H. Brookes Publishing Co.

Provencal, G. (1987) *Characteristics of a Successful Community Living Program and Support Service*. Melbourne: Yungaburra Foundation.

Robertson, J., Emerson, E., Hatton, C., Elliott, J., McIntosh, B., Swift, P., Krinjen-Kemp, E., Towers, C., Romeo, R., Knapp, M., Sanderson, H., Routledge, M., Oakes, P. and Joyce, T. (2005) *The Impact of Person Centred Planning*. Lancaster: Institute for Health Research, Lancaster University.

Rudkin, A. and Rowe, D. (2001) 'Planning for life', *Learning Disability Practice*, 3(5): 22–6.

Smull, M. and Sanderson, H. (2005) *Essential Lifestyle Planning for Everyone*, Manchester: The Learning Community – Essential Lifestyle Planning.

Stone, K. (1999) *To Stand Beside: The Advocacy for Inclusion Manual*. St Abbotsford, Canberra: VIC Stone and Associates.

Useful resources

Families Leading Planning UK
www.familiesleadingplanning.co.uk

The Learning Community of Essential Lifestyle Planning
www.elpnet.net

Valuing People Support Team
www.valuingpeople.gov.uk

12 Support planning

Helen Sanderson and Simon Duffy

Key issues

- Self-directed support
- Support plans
- Individual budgets
- Individualisation
- Empowerment

Introduction

Person centred planning is fundamental to self-directed support. The development of individual budgets requires people to have a support plan. A support plan is the name for the plan that shows how someone's Individual Budget will be spent, and the foundation of support planning is person centred planning. Indeed, support planning can be seen as person centred planning when you know the resources you are entitled to use.

In this chapter we describe the relationship between care plans and support plans, the role of care managers and professionals in support planning, explore the key elements of a support plan, and the role of professionals in developing support plans and reviewing plans.

Background and context

In the past 15 years at least, there have been two significant policy developments within health and social care. One trend has been to encourage professionals to make their interventions more individualised. The second has been to encourage people to take more control over their own lives. We might call the first trend individualisation and the second empowerment. Obviously these are similar trends, but they are not identical.

One field where both these trends can be identified is the activity of planning. It has been common for government and professional bodies to encourage more individualised planning just as there has been a rhetorical shift away from providing standardised or depersonalised forms of support or care. Individualised planning was critical to the Community Care reforms of the early 1990s (Department of Health 1989) and to later policies such as the development of the Care Programme Approach (Department of Health 1995).

However, there has always been an ongoing tension between the centralised desire for individualisation and the means of achieving it. It appears that once government has decided that professionals must be more individualised in their responses, they struggle to identify effective means to change professional behaviour and in some respects government seems to exacerbate the problem, both directly and indirectly, by inconsistent measures.

Recent initiatives like the development of the Single Assessment Process and the development of the Common Assessment Framework (Department of Health 2001) represent attempts to impose common structures on the planning process. Imposing a common structure is undertaken even before anyone is satisfied that any particular local structure is out-performing the others in encouraging individualised solutions. In the light of these initiatives it is hard not to see the promotion of individualised planning as a rhetorical device rather than as a clear and well-understood part of government policy.

However, there has been a second path to individualisation. In particular, we have seen the disability movement help people to achieve independent living with disabled people controlling their lives and their support (Gillinson et al. 2005). There have also been examples of good professional practice, for example, the promotion of genuine supported living for people with learning difficulties (Kinsella 1993). These forms of practice have not been imposed by government but have flowed from local initiatives, from leaders within the disability community or even from social entrepreneurs. What these initiatives share is the realisation that true individualisation can only be effective when the disabled person is no longer treated as a passive recipient of professional help. Instead people must have the power to shape their own lives, including when people may also need significant help in some or all aspects of their life.

This second trend, the shift to empowerment, is seen in the activity of planning in a number of ways. Person centred planning is an example of empowering planning. Research shows that person centred planning contributes to people having more choice in their lives, being more involved in their community, and having more contact with friends and family.

Activity 12.1

What challenges do you think individualisation and empowerment will present for professionals working within services?

In principle, these two trends should be mutually supportive. Strengthening the voice of the person as they engage with professional services should not conflict with strengthening the capacity of professionals to listen carefully and offer individualised interventions. However, in reality, they have rubbed against each other in a number of ways and for several interconnected reasons:

1   Currently care managers (or others) are expected to tailor a care plan to meet the needs of the individual. The system expectation is that it is the professional who controls and produces the plan and often such plans are constrained by standardised formats.
2   Even if a professional is willing in principle to treat a self-assessment or person centred plan as an adequate alternative to a professional care plan, the disabled person still has no knowledge of what resources might be available. Hence their own plans may vary widely in realism and affordability and are less likely to be acceptable when seeking resources from the professional system.
3   The real, but unspoken, currency of the care management process is the service options that have already been pre-purchased by the local authority and the options that are already treated as conventional and acceptable services to purchase. Hence, any plan that does not rely on 'typical services' is unlikely to be accepted.
4   Person centred planning tends to use family, friends and community as a natural source of support and inspiration when planning. Yet the strong involvement of others, outside of the disabled person, is highly problematic for many professional practices. Person centred planning challenges the tendency of existing professional practice to treat the relationship between the disabled person and the professional as the dominant relationship and the tendency to treat others as sources of either interference or abuse.
5   Finally, current rationing practice tends to take support from family and friends for granted and the system aims to only fund support that cannot be provided in this way. This is an incentive for family and friends to tactically withdraw from offering support – in order to generate an entitlement to support for the person they care about. This also makes it very difficult to produce an honest person centred

plan 'for services' for a plan that is rich with unpaid support that will be a poor tool for negotiating for resources.

In effect, the current structure of power and organisation within the delivery of social care has created a seemingly unbridgeable chasm with the process of professional assessment and care planning on one side and person centred planning, led by the person and their allies, on the other (see Figure 12.1).

It is the aim of this chapter to explore how this chasm can be bridged and to describe how the concept of a support plan can be used to reconcile these two different approaches to planning. We will do so by describing the work of the in Control programme and its model of self-directed support (Poll et al. 2006).

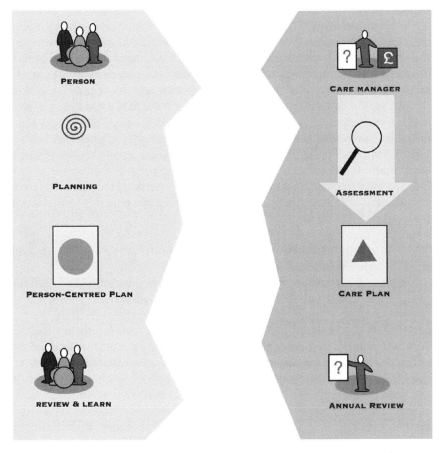

Figure 12.1   The social care chasm
Source: Reproduced with kind permission of in Control

In Control and self-directed support

In Control was launched in 2003 to begin developing a coherent and universal system of self-directed support to replace the current social care system. It began by piloting a model of self-directed support in six local authorities and, in 2005 it began working on a wider basis. By the middle of 2007 more than 90 local authorities had joined in Control and were working on promoting self-directed support, to some degree or other. The early indications are that this new way of working has successfully combined a more empowering and effective approach with better use of existing resources (Robertson et al. 2005).

The hypothesis that in Control tested was that the fundamental balance of power in the present social care system could be altered, significantly, through coherent system change. This shift in approach can be represented as a shift from the professional gift model to the citizenship model (see Chapter 4 for more information). This power shift involves taking as a starting point the right of the disabled person to direct their own life, and to do so with the support and help of their community. State-funded support should no longer be received as an unpredictable 'gift' but should become a transparent entitlement, enabling the individual to take charge of it and to use those resources flexibly in the context of their whole life. Professionals are no longer gate keepers, instead they are accountable to disabled people. Their services are only used when they are valued. This fundamental shift in power and structure is still under way and is highly contentious, involving, as it does, considerable economic and social change.

At a more detailed level in Control also had to respond to the need to have a coherent account of how planning should take place in this new system. It was faced with two realities:

- Planning must be person centred: it must serve the interests and preferences of the disabled person.
- Local authorities must be assured that there is an individual plan for the person and that it must be of a suitable quality.

Given these two realities, in Control's solution was both simple but radical. Within in Control's model of best practice – which local authorities can adopt – it is now possible for the individual to use their own plan as evidence to the local authority that a plan informs their support. In this instance it is not problematic for planning to be genuinely person centred for there is no 'competing' care plan to be completed by a professional. The local authority's need to assure itself that any such plan is adequate is met by declaring in advance what the criteria for success would be within the support plan. This allows care management to refocus their efforts on evaluating and agreeing the plans proposed by the person.

To put the point crudely, a support plan replaces the need for a care plan; a support plan is developed by the person with help where necessary, and it describes how the person intends to be supported in order to live their own life. The word 'support' is used in preference to 'care' because the verb 'support' is always an auxiliary verb, it is support to do something and so it implies that support is there to help people achieve their goals and ambitions. The word 'care' is very different, there is no natural implication that the person is actively involved – we can even 'care' for 'things'.

However, this shift from 'care plan' to 'support plan' involves much more than a change in the use of language. Critically the support plan is possible because of four critical innovations. These innovations are designed to bridge the chasm between the professionally-led process and the person centred process (see Figure 12.2).

The first innovation was the use of an individual budget, or an indicative allocation, which is provided on the basis of an early and relatively quick assessment of needs and against open and fair rules of entitlement. In Control has developed a number of ways of making such an indicative allocation and these are documented in detail elsewhere (see www.in-control.org.uk). The impact of this early and indicative allocation is vital to enable people to overcome both the lack of realistic constraints and the disincentive to build community into the current system as described above.

The second innovation was to reposition the role of the care manager, not as the necessary author of the plan, but as a facilitator and possible supporter. Support from the care manager should be proportional to the need for that support and there is strong evidence, not least from care managers themselves, that they are not always necessarily involved in the support planning and that other individuals or professionals may be better able to support the process of detailed planning.

The third key innovation was to change the care manager's role into offering a critical evaluation of the plans proposed by individuals. Instead of being the presumed expert on the disabled person (arguably a near impossible role for any professional to be asked to play), the care manager is expected to be a critical friend – ensuring that the person has not forgotten to consider key issues or made unrealistic assumptions. This new role is not only both more realistic and more useful to the disabled person, it is also more likely to enable the local authority to better meet its own duty of care to the disabled person.

The final innovation was to rethink the review process, which is a necessary component of the care management process, but a component that has become increasingly marginalised over recent years. Instead of treating the care manager as an 'inspector' of services, the focus shifts to requiring the disabled person to be accountable and to share what they have learnt from the process of being in control. Instead of thinking in terms of the adequacy of a

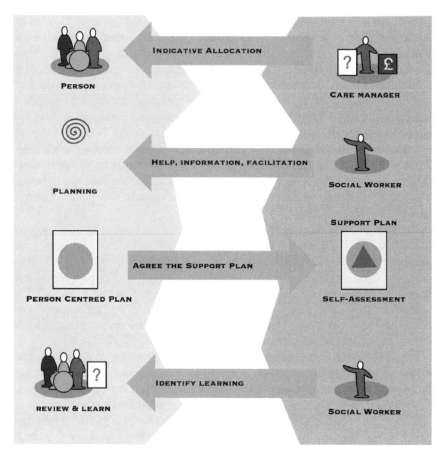

Figure 12.2 Bridging the social care chasm
Source: Reproduced with kind permission of in Control

placement – a fixed service into which the person must fit – the care manager has a positive role in helping the disabled person keep control of their life and make any necessary changes.

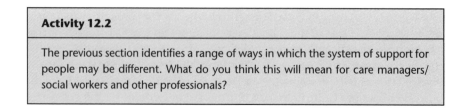

Activity 12.2

The previous section identifies a range of ways in which the system of support for people may be different. What do you think this will mean for care managers/ social workers and other professionals?

A different role for professionals

The changes identified in the previous section indicate what will be necessary to change the way that people will work. All professionals will need to move to a position of listening to what other people are saying to them about what is important *to* them and *for* them, and identify ways that they can offer their expertise to people in a way that is acceptable to them. Professionals will become experts for people to refer to, rather than experts about people.

Gerry Smale (1993) offers a useful analysis of these different approaches to care management assessment and care planning that can also provide insight into the ways in which a range of professionals operate, as can be seen in Box 12.1.

Box 12.1 Different models of professional care

Questioning model	In the questioning model, the care manager/professional asks questions to determine what the person needs. The questions reflect what the professional sees as important according to their particular expertise, and understanding of 'need'. The person's disability and its impact on their life are typically the focus of the questions. This approach assumes that professional knowledge provides the critical authority for the care manager's or other professional's work and this authority is exercised as a professional judgement about the individual's needs.
Procedural model	The second possible approach is the procedural model; in this model the critical authority for the care manager's work is the system of services and resources that are available for the disabled person. Instead of exercising professional judgement, the care manager has a set of forms to complete to determine the person's eligibility for these services. The professional's expertise is used to accurately complete the forms and determine action. The care manager is effectively an agent of the statutory authority, operating with limited discretion to ensure the objectivity of the decisions that are made, offering statutory authorities a seemingly fair and efficient way of rationing and allocating resources. From the perspective of other professional groups' the rationing and application of pre-determined resources may also be of relevance.
Exchange model	In the exchange model it is assumed that the person is the expert in their life and problems, and that professional expertise lies in helping to create a shared understanding of the person and their situation, negotiating, problem solving and co-designing solutions. Smale (1993) states: '*It is assumed that all people are expert in their own problems and that there is no reason to assume that the worker will or should ever know more about people and their problems than they do themselves, and certainly not before they do.*'

As indicated in the work of Smale, significant challenges face many professions but nowhere will the changes be more significant than for care managers and social workers. The following section focuses particularly upon this group of people.

A different role for care managers and social workers

Both the questioning and procedural models of care management are prevalent and highly unattractive. Both models radically limit the ability of the individual to take control of their own lives; moreover, both models fail to respect the genuine and positive contribution that care managers can make. It is only the exchange model that offers an attractive account of the process of care management in self-directed support.

The principles of self-directed support challenge both the questioning and procedural models. The paternalist assumptions of the past are being replaced by an increased understanding that people have rights, including a right to self-determination. Services are no longer seen as an unmitigated good, to be parcelled out by benevolent professionals. Instead individuals, families and professionals are recognising that they must work in the spirit of the exchange model, by collaboration.

What all this means is that the shift from support planning to care planning is not primarily a question of changing terminology or paperwork. The fundamental shift is in the role played by the care manager and the different relationship that they will have with the disabled person. In particular, their role is likely to become more focused on:

- Review and problem solving, instead of assessment and care planning. Arguably this offers us a way back to the heart of social work and reflects the 'exchange model' way of working.
- Working with people in particularly complex situations, perhaps where the person has lost the support of family and friends or where they are subject to abuse from services or from individuals.

The care manager has a unique contribution to make, to enable people to reflect on their progress, on what has worked well and the challenges they have encountered, and to work with people to plan their next steps. Care managers are in a good position to make the following contributions (see Box 12.2).

In the rest of this chapter we will set out the implications of this new approach to planning and care management and some of the early lessons and areas for further exploration. In particular, we will explore how support planning works in practice, the qualities of an effective support plan, who can help develop support plans, what helps support planning and the important area of reviewing plans.

Box 12.2 Skills and knowledge of care managers	
Systems knowledge	Care managers are well positioned to help the individual navigate the human service system itself: the rules, policies and procedures, the various service options and the systems of advocacy, complaint and conciliation. The care manager is in the ideal position to deliver this information.
Review and action planning skills	Reflection and planning are central to the job of the care manager, enabling them to facilitate good decision-making by the individual and those close to them at the review stage of the process.
Community knowledge	Good support does not just involve using professional services it also involves using community resources: relationships and friendships, employers, associations and groups, leisure and ordinary community facilities and many other aspects of ordinary life. Again, care managers will not be the only people who know about these resources, but care managers may have their own knowledge of the community to enable people to plan the next steps after reviewing progress.
Individual insight	While each of us may be a relative expert on our own needs and while the people close to us may know us better than the people who are more distant, there is always room for individual insight. Sometimes someone different can see something different. Knowledge of the self and knowledge of our needs are always imperfect and there is no reason why even a stranger cannot contribute their own insights.

How does support planning work in practice?

There are seven steps to being in control, and these are summarised in Box 12.3. The first step is where the person finds out how much money they are likely to receive, and then they plan how to spend that, by developing a support plan. The support plan is agreed in step 3, and then put into practice in steps 4, 5 and 6. The review process in step 7 enables people to reflect and learn and then plan further actions by updating or recreating their support plan.

Box 12.3 The seven steps to being in control	
1 Self-assessment	Find out how much money they are likely to be able to receive – called the *Individual Budget*.
2 Plan support	Work out how they should use that money to meet their needs in a way that suits them best. This is recorded in a support plan.

3 Agree the plan	Check out their *Assessment and Support Plan* with the local authority or any other funder. This is where the support plan is agreed.
4 Manage individual budget	Find the best way for them to manage their *Individual Budget*.
5 Organise support	Organise the housing, help, equipment or other kinds of things to get their life going well.
6 Live life	Use their support to live a full life with family and friends in their community.
7 Review and learn	Check out that things are going OK and make changes if they need to.

What are the qualities of an effective support plan?

Support planning is a process for thinking about the person's life, what they want to change, and how they will use their individual budget to make those changes. As suggested earlier, support plans can and should replace care plans where people have individual budgets. As with person centred plans, support plans can be written in different ways. They may be short or long – with pictures or just text. The person can write it for themselves or have someone else write it for them. One of the differences between support plans and person centred plans, is that a support plan has to fulfil certain criteria to be signed off by a care manager, including a financial cost for the support the person intends to have. Further details about what constitutes an effective support plan and what does not can be found at www.in-control.org.uk or www.supportplanning.org

In summary, however, this means that a support plan should be as shown in Table 12.1.

Table 12.1 Features of a good support plan

Feature required	Definition
Person centred	It must suit you and fit your preferred lifestyle.
Clear	You should set yourself clear and meaningful outcomes to achieve.
Practical	You should know how you will achieve your outcomes.
Safe	You should make sure you and others are not put unnecessarily at risk.
Self-determined	You should be in as much control of decisions as possible.
Managed	You need clear systems of management and responsibility.
In budget	You must not spend more than the agreed income.

Reviewing and signing off plans are part of key training for care managers and social workers. In some areas this takes place at a panel, for example, in one authority they test plans at a risk enablement panel, so far, while some plans have been modified, none have been refused by the panel.

Who can help people write support plans?

Local authorities are responsible for ensuring that people get any help that they need to put together their support plan. Currently there are five ways of producing a plan:

1   People can complete it themselves.
2   People can complete it with support from friends and family.
3   People can complete it with support from the local authority.
4   People can purchase the support from an independent person, or people.
5   People can have a plan completed on their behalf – by any of the people in 2, 3 or 4.

Some people will simply work from the criteria to create their own way of putting together a support plan – the 'kitchen table approach'. Others may want more guidance, and will use person centred planning or any of the associated tools. Person centred planning usually involves the person getting together with their family and friends to develop a plan with the help of a person centred planning facilitator. Finally, some people will choose to have someone else create the support plan for them, under their direction (for further information, see www.supportplanning.org).

There are, therefore, a number of different people who could help:

- *Friends and family*: some people find it helpful to organise the people around them into a Trust – often called a 'Trust Circle'. This is a legal entity that is not difficult to set up. A Trust is particularly helpful where people need support in making decisions, or need people to sometimes make decisions on their behalf.
- *Service providers*: if people are already connected to an organisation that they trust and are happy with, then they could ask the organisation to help. Support workers, workers from a community group, or supported living organisations are some of the people who might help.

> *Margaret had been in hospital for sixty years and had no family or friends, she was not even liked by the ward staff. When she left*

hospital to live in her own home, her team formed a circle around her, connecting her to their family and friends. Margaret spent the last years of her life surrounded by love and affection with a team who really listened hard to what she wanted.

- *Person centred planning facilitators*: most areas now have trained person centred planning facilitators, including families and people who have a learning disability. In one authority they used a team of person centred planning facilitators working in partnership with care managers to develop support plans.
- *Care managers or social worker* (sometimes called care co-ordinators): some people may want their care manager to help them in developing their support plan.
- *People who are independent and would be paid to help someone in developing their support plan*: independent people may be able to help with some or all of the plan. For example, a life coach or person centred planning facilitator could help someone think about the changes they want to make, while a financial advisor could help work out the budget for implementing the plan.

Kenny already knew Tony well – he had been his friend and advocate for many years. Together they wrote Kenny's support plan, describing the life that Kenny wanted to live, away from St Johns in Devon, and back to Essex.

These independent people include: Centres for Independent Living; support brokers; independent advocates; Direct Payments support schemes; independent person centred planning facilitators; life coaches; Financial advisors; and other people or organisations that the person knows and trusts.

It is important to develop a mixed approach when developing your vision for support planning. People need to be able to choose from several options rather than solely relying, for example, on care managers or support brokers.

Support planning and person centred planning

As support planning is part of the family of person centred planning, the results of the research into the impact of person centred planning (Robertson et al. 2005) can be applied here. The most significant finding relating to the success of person centred planning was the commitment of the facilitator to the values of person centred planning (i.e. the values of inclusion). Therefore we could infer from this that one of the significant factors that people could consider when choosing someone to help them plan, is their commitment and understanding of the values of self-directed support and inclusion. It is also very helpful if people and those enabling them to develop their support plans have a wide variety of examples of different ways people could use their money for support.

For example, instead of using money to buy three days at a day centre, someone could buy SKY TV, or gym membership and three hours paid support from someone to accompany them. Or they could pay for community transport to go to, say, Centre Parcs to join their extended family on holiday.

It is too early to provide an authoritative picture of the different ways in which support planning will be provided. However, some early work with care managers was suggestive of the possibilities. At a series of independent sessions, care managers (mostly, but not exclusively, working with people with learning difficulties) were asked to identify real people in their case loads and then to decide, from their knowledge of the person and their situation, who would be the best to develop a support plan for the individual. Figure 12.3 sets out the distribution of 803 people and the care manager's view of who would be the best person to lead the development of the support plan.

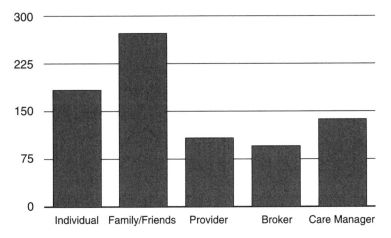

Figure 12.3   Care manager's view of best option for development of support plan
Source: Reproduced with kind permission of in Control

The impact of a mixed economy of support planning on the role and function of care managers

This data is the result of a hypothetical exercise. Nevertheless it is interesting because it represents the views of the one group who might be said to have a vested interest in over-estimating their own relative importance. Yet what this data suggests is that care managers themselves can identify many people where the best leadership for support planning comes from else-where. Moreover they do not think that there is always one best person to lead the process of support planning, but that good person centred planning might be led or supported by different kinds of people in different circumstances.

If this analysis is correct, it implies a significant change in the role of those who are currently care managers. But not a simple or unidimensional shift in role. If we were to apply this analysis to current data about the actual workload of care managers, then a number of possible changes can be identified. For example, if we analyse the finding of the report, 'What do care managers do?' (Weinberg et al. 2003), then this suggests that currently the balance of care management workload is as follows:[1]

> First Point of Contact – 6.8 per cent
> Assessment Information – 27.0 per cent
> Planning Support – 2.4 per cent
> Developing Support – 7.6 per cent
> Problem solving – 11.3 per cent
> Reviewing – 4.4 per cent
> Organisational Functions – 40.5 per cent

If we were then to convert the care management system over to self-directed support, we might expect the following reductions in workload:

- Significant reduction in time spent on gathering assessment infor-mation, because the setting of an indicative allocation usually requires a very minimal first assessment of need.
- Also, according to the data above, development of the support plan should be led by others in 83 per cent of cases.
- There may also be some increase in the level of service development carried out by individuals, families or other professionals under self-directed support.

However, this reduction will most likely be balanced by:

- Much more attention being paid to the review process to ensure people are well and that the particular arrangement for self-directed support is working.
- Much more detailed person centred planning being done for those (17 per cent) who really require significant help from their care managers to plan.

These changes are only at an early stage. Only a few care management teams are using self-directed support as the default system at this stage. Furthermore it is likely that inherited practices will need to be thoughtfully revisited before a significant rebalancing of role could take place. The inherited culture of care management will tend to discourage the necessary trust in individuals, families or friends, or even other professionals. Self-directed support creates the opportunity for change, but only local leadership by care managers can make the change real. Nevertheless change is possible (see Box 12.4).

Box 12.4 Michael's support plan

Michael lives at home with his Mum and Dad. He hated going to the day centre and wanted more personal assistance and the opportunity to have some more independence within the family home. His care manager arrived and discussed his needs and suggested that a package of £30,000 per year (which included £20,000 from the ILF) would be available to Michael. The family were also left a short description of what needed to be in the support plan. The following week the care manager returned and received a support plan including the financial costs from the family. Michael, his parents, his brother and his sister-in-law had met for Sunday lunch and developed the plan. The care manager admitted that it would have taken her several months to complete the normal assessment and care plan and that this would have been no better than what the family had done themselves. The plan was agreed almost immediately and within a few weeks the new support was in place.

Ultimately this shift in role may not be the creation of a new role for care managers, rather it may mean the return to values and practices that were always part of social work. As Andrew Tyson, a social worker and commissioner in West Sussex says:

> *This will mean, for some, a welcome return to 'traditional social work'. But for others it will mean new and unfamiliar ways of working with people, and a move away from what 'care management' has come to mean. For all, it is important to be clear how social workers are now being asked to work with disabled people and families.*

What can help people to make a support plan?

Whoever is helping the person to develop their support plan, whether this is a professional, family member or person centred planning facilitator, there are a range of processes and materials available.

Materials

One of the big challenges is to make sure that a new system of self-directed support does not end up as complicated or as dependent upon specialists and experts as the old system. The system must be easy to use, one that all citizens can navigate around, as much as possible and with as little interference as possible.

There are a number of guides developed that are based on person centred planning and directly relate to the criteria for signing off plans. These guides are designed to enable people to develop support plans, and include 'In the Driving Seat', for people with learning disabilities and their allies. This is accompanied by 'Top Tips' which gives examples and suggestions for people who are using 'In the Driving Seat'. Some people prefer to use a graphic rather than solely a text-based process. There are several template versions available that cover the information required for the support plan to be signed off (Figure 12.4).

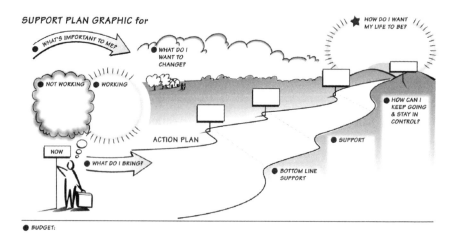

Figure 12.4 Support plan graphic
Source: Reprinted with kind permission from Helen Sanderson Associates

Person centred planning

In practice, person centred planning provides an excellent basis for a support plan. Caroline used a 'PATH' to begin to create Joe's support plan:

> *Joe already had a circle of friends. The circle consisted of people who loved and cared about Joe and other people who were paid to be in his life. The social worker also came and used these meetings as a starting point for his assessment. At the circle meeting we used a person centred planning process called 'PATH' to think about Joe's dreams and visions for the future, what his skills and gifts were, a step-by-step approach to how he was going to get there and who we needed to involve.*

Each of the person centred planning processes involved getting people together to explore issues and agree actions. Person centred planning and support planning can also be done in small groups, with people working simultaneously on their plans. This process is called Planning Live.

Planning Live

This process can take place over two or three days, depending on the pace that would work best for people, their access needs and degree of comfort.

These are the key ingredients for 'Planning Live':

- People know what their resource allocation is, and any restrictions to how they can use their individual budget.
- People can come with someone who will support them (for example, their support planner, care manager, family member or independent broker).
- People can invite other people to come and help them as well if they choose (for example, partners, family, friends).
- The day is led by a trainer (two for a group of more than four people with their supporters).
- The two or three days can be split over two weeks or more, to give people time to add to their plans or talk to other people if necessary.

People sit at tables with their supporter and any other people that they have invited. The trainer will work with a volunteer at the front, and explain and demonstrate with the volunteer how each question can be approached. People then work on the question themselves. Then the trainer and volunteer explain and demonstrate the second question, and everyone then has a go at that, and so on. The trainer works at the pace of the group, and goes round each table to assist as necessary. Some people choose to use a graphic template to record their support plan, others prefer to write it (see Box 12.5).

Box 12.5 Donna's support plan

Donna attended training days which were held in a community hall in Bristol at the weekend. Donna had the opportunity to talk about her support needs and think about plans for her future. Following on from this, Donna attended more meetings where she worked in small groups with others to talk about her plans for life and as a result came away with the start of her plan! Donna says she was very nervous at first when thinking about plans for the future but as she went along became more familiar with different ideas and felt much more confident in making decisions. Over the next few months Donna wrote plans and started to make decisions about her future.

Planning Live has been used successfully in Essex, where they are now building local capacity to develop this with disabled people as trainers. This is what some of the first 'Individual Budgeteers' have told us about their experiences of Planning Live with Individual Budgets:

> *Personally I have had a great mistrust of social services, my goal is to be as independent as possible. I found the whole experience fulfilling – the people I thought were in control were suddenly with me. There was less of a feeling of them and us, this time it was like we are in it together.*

For more information about planning live, see *www.supportplanning.org*

Reviewing support plans

Once support plans have been agreed and signed off, they are reviewed with the care manager annually. The review process is the key to ensuring that we hear about the changes people are making in their life, how they are using their money, and what they have discovered on this journey. It is about learning, change and accountability, not audit. The process is a natural extension of support planning. The review process reflects the questions used for signing off support plans. Care managers or budget holders expect plans to clearly communicate what is important to you, what you want to change, how you will be supported, how you will spend your money and manage your support, how you will stay in control and what you are going to do next. In the review process, we take the same issues and address them under four headings:

'living your life', 'spending your budget', 'staying in control of your life' and 'getting and managing your support'.

For many people this is the heart of social work – supporting people to review their progress, problem solve and plan next steps, and this is a crucial role for care managers in the individual budget process. The following approach is suggested for conducting reviews.

Review questions '4 plus 2'

The process that we want people to use is called the '4 plus 2' questions. The four questions ask what people have tried, learned, are pleased about or concerned about in relation to four areas of their life (Figure 12.5). The areas are:

1   *Living your life*. By this we mean that people have what is important to them in their life, and have been able to change what they were dissatisfied with.
2   *Spending your budget*. What people have tried in relation to money. This is not an audit, this is an opportunity for people to say how they used their budget (for some people this will differ from what they planned to do in their support plan) and what this means for how they want to use their money in the future.
3   *Staying in control of your life*. This will mean exploring the different ways that people have found to stay in control of their lives and their support.
4   *Getting and managing your support*. Identifying how their natural and paid support has worked out for them.

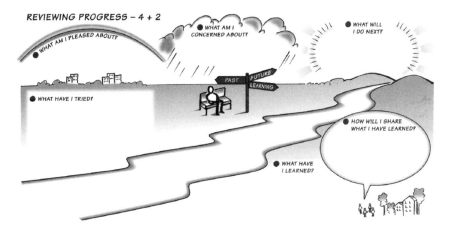

Figure 12.5   Reviewing progress – 4 plus 2
Source: Reprinted with kind permission from Helen Sanderson Associates

The 'Plus 2' questions relate to what people are going to do next, and how to share what they have learned.

What will you do next?

People may come with clear ideas about what they want to stay the same and what they want to change, where this is not the case, the person's support or the care manager could help them think about this. The review should end with an action plan of next steps.

How can we share what you have learned?

There is an expectation that learning is shared, in a way that works for the person. The care manager or whoever is leading the review is responsible for helping people to think about what they want to share and the best way to do this. The care manager will have a prompt list to think through with the person about what, where and how their learning can be shared.

Sharing learning

Each review should result in shared learning. We want to be able to spot innovations to share and inspire, identify the traps to avoid, and practical solutions to common problems. Learning can be shared at a peer, local and national level.

Sharing learning at a peer level

Decisions in this area should be informed by the following questions/ suggestions:

- What would other disabled people find useful? Example support plans? Local contacts that provided a great service? Ways around difficulties and problems?
- What is the best way to share this? For example, Centres for Independent Living news letter, information on local website, example plans on websites?

Sharing learning at a local level

Decisions in this area should be informed by the following questions/ suggestions:

- Who would benefit from hearing this? Who are our local stakeholders in the community and services? How can this inform the local commissioning strategy? What does this tell us about what needs to change in the way we are developing systems for self-directed support?

- What is the best way to share this information? How can it get to the self-directed support/in Control steering/management group? Would it be useful to place information in a local paper? GP surgery?

Sharing learning at a national level
Decisions in this area should be informed by the following questions/ suggestions:

- Who would benefit from hearing this nationally? For example, the CSIP implementation team? In Control Board and Core Team? National press?
- What is the best way to share this information? For example, through the local lead person? Through the Communications Director of in Control?

Whatever the decisions in relation to the above areas, it is important to share information that will be useful to the continued development of this new innovation in supporting people to have the lives that they want.

One of the first care managers to use this approach to reviews said: '*Over the last few years I have been looking for a review process that is meaningful to people – this is it.*' For more information on the approach to reviews, see www.in-control.org.uk Information within this section is reproduced with kind permission of in Control.

Conclusion

Where people have an individual budget, support planning is replacing care planning. Rooted in the principles underpinning person centred planning, support planning represents four critical innovations. The first is individual budgets where people can plan from a position of knowing what money they are entitled to. The second innovation repositions the role of the care manager from the person who writes care plans to someone who ensures that people have any assistance that they need to develop their support plan. The third innovation also relates to the role of the care manager, in ensuring that support plans meet the relevant criteria. Finally, the fourth innovation concerns the review process which is critical in enabling people to be accountable and for sharing learning.

For many care managers, this represents a return 'to the heart of social work'. For others this will require a change in thinking and practice, to perform new roles that enable disabled people to live the lives they choose.

Note

1   The analysis of Weinberg et al. is a very detailed task-focused analysis. To arrive at the analysis given here Simon Duffy mapped those tasks against the core functions of care management. This data was from services for older people and clearly it would be a mistake to treat these figures as offering a precise of universal account of the current balance of the care management function. Nevertheless, we hope the figures provide sufficient sense of the current reality to enable us to begin to imagine the possible impact of Self-Directed Support upon the care management function.

Annotated bibliography

Duffy, S. (2006) *Keys to Citizenship*, 2nd edn. Birkenhead: Paradigm.
This book is a guide for anyone who wants to develop individual services for people with learning difficulties. It offers practical advice covering all the main topics that should be considered when helping someone with a learning difficulty plan for their future: Self-determination, Direction, Money, Home, Support and Community Life. The book includes stories of innovation and success as well as a step-by-step guide on matters such as finding a job, buying a house and making friends. In an easy to read style, it is suitable for anyone who wants to make practical changes in their own life or in the life of someone they care about.

Poll, C., Duffy, S., Hatton, C., Sanderson, H. and Routledge, M. (2006) *A Report on in Control's First Phase 2003–2005*. London: in Control Publications.
This is a report from the first two years of in Control. This report describes the model and evaluation, phase one, of in Control in detail along with stories and learning from the first six sites.

References

Department of Health (1989) *Caring for People*. London: HMSO.
Department of Health (1995) *Building Bridges: A Guide to Arrangements for Inter-agency Working for the Care and Protection of Severely Mentally Ill People*. London: HMSO.
Department of Health (2001) *National Service Framework for Older People*. London: Department of Health.
Duffy, S. (2006) *Keys to Citizenship*, 2nd edn. Birkenhead: Paradigm.
Gillinson, S., Green, H. and Miller, P. (2005) *Independent Living: The Right to be Equal Citizens*. London: Demos.

Kinsella, P. (1993) *Supported Living: A New Paradigm*. Manchester: NDT.

Poll, C., Duffy, S., Hatton, C., Sanderson, H. and Routledge, M. (2006) *A Report on in Control's First Phase 2003–2005*. London: in Control Publications.

Robertson, J., Emerson, E., Hatton, C., Elliott, J., McIntosh, B., Swift, P., Krinjen-Kemp, E., Towers, C., Romeo, R., Knapp, M., Sanderson, H., Routledge, M., Oakes, P. and Joyce, T. (2005) *The Impact of Person Centred Planning*. Lancaster: Institute for Health Research, Lancaster University.

Smale, G. (1993) *Empowerment, Assessment, Care Management and the Skilled Worker*. London: HMSO.

Weinberg, A., Williamson, J., Challis, D. and Hughes, J. (2003) What do care managers do? A study of working practice in older peoples' services, *British Journal of Social Work*, 33: 901–19.

Useful resources

Helen Sanderson Associates
www.helensandersonassociates.co.uk

in Control website
www.in-control.org.uk

Support Planning Website
www.supportplanning.org

13 Creating community inclusion

Jo Kennedy, Carl Poll and Helen Sanderson

Key issues

- What is community?
- Barriers to community
- Approaches to building community
- The role of professionals in building community
- Practical approaches to helping people to engage in their community
- Strategic community building examples

Introduction

In society there is a sense that we have lost 'community' and that this is endemic across the Western world. When we say this, we are referring to the growth of communities that are derived from competitive and highly industrial societies in which relationships are not an end in themselves but more a means to profit and self-interest. This is a community in which personal involvements are often superficial, calculating and impersonal. This is in contrast to the communities we would like to see that are typified by a sense of intimacy, face-to-face relationships and a sense of belonging. The message of this chapter is that one way to reinvigorate community as we would like to conceptualise it is to put an end to the exclusion of disabled people and older people from making their contribution.

Professionals have an important role in achieving this as people with learning disabilities often need to be encouraged and supported to assert their rights as citizens. One key way to achieve this is by supporting people to use mainstream support and funding to access their community and influence services. In this chapter we will consider the professionals' role in a range of approaches to developing community. We begin by exploring the term 'community' and identifying the barriers that exist for people with learning disabilities to be fully included. We then examine the different approaches that professionals can take to support people to overcome these barriers.

'Community' – what do we mean?

According to Baldwin (1993), cited in Jones (1998), community is our endless connections with and responsibilities towards each other. Remarkably, for a word that is constantly in use, there is no consensus over what we mean by community, instead we have at least 94 different definitions. What there is a consensus on, is that society has lost a sense of 'community'. Putnam (2001) described this as a decline in 'social capital', the connections among individuals, social networks and the norms of reciprocity and trustworthiness which arise from these connections.

The concept of community can be explored by considering its component parts as described by Lee and Newby (1983):

- community as geography;
- community as a local social system;
- community as a shared identity.

In this chapter we concentrate less on community as geography and more on the latter two areas, community as a social system and as a shared identity including community as a place or a sense of belonging.

When we speak of community, we speak of belonging either to a neighbourhood, a network of family or friends or to a community of shared interest. This has been described as the sense that each of us is part of a readily available, mutually supportive network of relationships upon which we are able to depend and as a result of which, we do not experience sustained feelings of loneliness that impel a person to actions or to adapting to a lifestyle, masking anxiety and setting the stage for later more destructive anguish.

Activity 13.1	
What does community mean to you?	

For many people, community means their local neighbourhood, or a group or club they belong to. For others, it could be a group who share values as well as interests. However you define community, we know that there are barriers which prevent people with learning disabilities from being included in their community. It is the intention of this next section to discuss some of these barriers in more detail.

The barriers to community

The barriers to community exist within the community itself, within individuals with learning disabilities, in services and within government policy. Some of them are outlined below:

Within the community

Fear/hostility/prejudice: there is still discrimination against people with learning disabilities in the community and a lack of recognition that people with learning disabilities are entitled to the same rights and opportunities as every other member of society.

They are other people's problem: for as long as most people can remember, people with learning disabilities have been cared for by the state. This has fostered a belief in many people, including families, that they are not capable of talking to people with learning disabilities, let alone supporting them. This attitude extends to mainstream services and community organisations. Community development workers and community leaders, who have skills and experience in connecting people, often believe that it is the job of specialist services to offer any kind of support to people with learning disabilities. In this way people with learning disabilities are denied the opportunity to take up their role as a citizen in a community (see also Chapter 4 for further information).

Within individuals themselves

Individual's lack of networks: many people with learning disabilities have lived in institutions – they may have lost touch with their family, had few opportunities to make friends and little experience of what a friend is. Those who have lived at home may have been sheltered from the community. As a result, they may have few skills in developing friendships as opposed to more formal caring relationships.

In services

Staff ignorance on how to access community: many staff do not live in the communities in which they work. If they do, they may be isolated themselves and have no idea of how to find out about what is going on or how to build productive relationships in the neighbourhood.

Staff ignorance on how to support relationship building: supporting individuals to meet others and develop friendships is a new role for some staff and many may not have skills in this area or be uncomfortable about using them.

Staff/carer fear of what might happen: there are risks inherent in meeting strangers. The fear of what might happen can prevent supporters of an individual from helping them to meet new people. Additionally, some staff can develop a very protective attitude towards the people they care for and resent others stepping in to support them or offer them different opportunities.

Institutional barriers, for example, registration, group living: some organisations have had to change their structure in order to accommodate the desire of people with learning disabilities to be independent ordinary members of the community. Group living and group resourcing have been shown to get in the way of building friendships with people outside of the house. Registration requirements mean that houses often do not look like homes.

In policy

Mixed policy messages: while there is a genuine policy commitment to inclusion for people with learning disabilities (Scottish Executive 2000; Department of Health 2001), there is also an increasing concern about risk. Many agencies supporting people with learning disabilities will prefer to protect their clients from meeting others, thereby protecting themselves from prosecution if things go wrong. At the same time they will insist on running police checks on new people in an individual's life, signalling from the start that it is not an ordinary friendship. Although care services are subject to government inspection, this will not normally include a review of their effectiveness in community connecting, conveying the message that they will not be penalised if they neglect this area of work.

Activity 13.2

Having considered the barriers outlined above what can professionals do to help people become valued members of their community?
    What first steps can you take in your job to help this to happen?

There are different approaches that professionals can take to address many of these barriers and enable people to take their places as full community citizens. Pioneers of the movement to promote more inclusive communities, in both the USA and Britain, have attempted to understand and break down some of these barriers. The next section will consider five of these approaches. These are:

1   The Inclusion Movement
2   Asset-based community development
3   The social model of disabilities

4   Community development
5   Active citizenship.

Approaches to building community

The first two of the above approaches were pioneered in North America and have been adapted for the UK context, the third is well established in much of the Western world and the fourth and fifth arise specifically out of the current UK context. It is our belief that each one can help overcome some of the barriers identified above, but to overcome all of them we need to work creatively with all five approaches, each of which has implications for the work of professionals. In this section we look at the five approaches, and identify how professionals can use each approach.

The inclusion movement

Judith Snow has developed a framework which maps relationships in four concentric circles (Figure 13.1). The inner circle, the circle of intimacy, is where those with whom we are closest, belong, our lover, husband or wife, our children, our dearest friends, those people who support us to define our

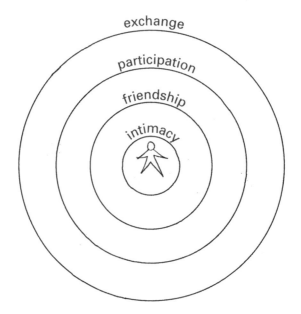

Figure 13.1   The circles of relationship
Source: Reprinted with kind permission from Kennedy et al. (2002)

identity. The second circle, the circle of friendship, includes good friends and less close family. The third circle, the circle of participation or membership, includes those people who belong to something with us. They may be work colleagues, or fellow members of a choir or church congregation, they could be neighbours or fellow students. The fourth circle, the circle of exchange is for those with whom we have a paid relationship – the hairdresser, the woman in the newsagent, the doctor, and so on.

One of the main points Judith draws from this analysis of relationships is that we need to be in a community to make friends. The people we meet at school or college, or at work or through the church are the people who become our friends and our lovers. People can move from the third circle into the second circle and the first circle, nor is it impossible for people to move further away from the centre or out of our circle altogether.

Judith Snow is also very clear that people with learning disabilities bring gifts to a community. As well as the obvious skills and talents they have, which have sometimes been overlooked, they bring the gift of themselves, their presence, their difference and the opportunity they offer others to interact with them and with each other because of them. One of the very first Circles of Support, as we now understand them, was formed around Judith. Judith benefited, in that it enabled her to move out of the institution in which she was then living. But those in the circle benefited too, not only from the relationship they had with her but also from the ways relationships developed with each other as they worked towards a common aim (Snow 1994).

Some people with learning disabilities have used circles of support for themselves and have made friends through taking part in activities. However, many people have been isolated too long to tackle this on their own. Particularly, progressive learning disability services use this approach in training programmes with staff, who then go on to support people who use their service to meet people through joining in with community life. Taking this 'person centred' approach can be very effective in tackling some of the barriers identified in the previous section, including an individual's lack of networks and fear and ignorance in the community. However, this approach does not really attempt to tackle the service or policy barriers identified.

Asset-based community development

McKnight (1997) has argued that services can, unintentionally, stand between a person with a learning disability and the community. He believes that support offered by services is support that in some cases would otherwise be offered by the community. The result being that ordinary community members begin to feel themselves unable to assist or even communicate with people with learning disabilities, believing that you need a special qualification to do so. Like Judith Snow, John McKnight believes that people with learning disabilities are not given the opportunity to show their assets to a community as they are always being assessed in terms of what is wrong with them. It is these 'gifts' that form the basis of the essential currency of community exchange. He advocates the stepping aside of services in order to allow people with learning disabilities to contribute to their community, and for people in the community to demonstrate their natural hospitality.

McKnight takes a community development approach to connecting people with learning disabilities to their communities. His method is to research all the formal and informal clubs and associations, from mother and toddler groups to Rotary Clubs, in a particular area. He believes that these associations offer the route to community for those who are excluded. Within those associations are people who believe in their community, who wish to welcome people into it, and are well connected themselves. These people he calls 'community guides'. And it is these people who can introduce those with learning disabilities into their community and find them opportunities to express their gifts.

Again, progressive learning disability services have drawn on these ideas, encouraging staff to draw up community maps, seek out 'community guides' and to support individuals to join local clubs and associations. In this way they try to counteract service and community barriers including staff ignorance of how to access the local community and fear in community members.

The work of both Judith Snow and John McKnight is rooted in the North American tradition of individual generosity and a healthy and independent associational life. It does not attempt to engage with the service or policy context in the UK. Although it provides energy and inspiration to people with learning disabilities, their friends and support staff, it ignores the local government structures, which could be used much more effectively to promote healthy communities.

The social model of disability

The social model of disability defines the problem of exclusion as societal rather than individual. Disability activists, working with allies, in Britain and the USA have focused on changing the structure of our society to enable disabled people to exercise their right to be included. The Disability Discrimination Act (2004) and the accessibility of cities like San Francisco are evidence of their success. But there are still many thousands of cinemas, restaurants, clubs, cafes and workplaces which disabled people are unable to access.

This model has had a clear influence on the emerging UK policy in relation to people with learning disabilities, which is increasingly based on a rights perspective and attempts to counteract discrimination against people with learning disabilities. It is a model that tackles policy barriers and is very useful in the context of staff training. However, in practice, people with learning disabilities themselves have to some extent been ignored in this debate. They are not always connected to or included in groups lobbying on behalf of disabled people and have set up separate self-advocacy groups like People First. In addition, this model focuses much more on societal rather than individual issues and does not in itself set out to help people develop their own personal networks. Its contribution is, however, invaluable in the wider context in which individual networks are developed.

Community development tradition

One of the factors which makes Britain distinct from the USA is the existence of mainstream statutory services which are dedicated to promoting healthy communities. Although it has been argued that some services block people from accessing their communities, the reverse is also true. Good services, which are really based on community development principles, can also be a great asset in working towards inclusion.

In Britain, there is a strong tradition of community development. The Scottish Community Development Centre has produced a model of community development that is based on research with practitioners in the field and has been widely accepted as good practice (see Figure 13.2).

A healthy community has the following key characteristics:

- It is liveable, for instance, a place or a social network within which people's needs are met, where they feel comfortable and have a sense of belonging.
- It is sustainable, for instance, in social, environmental and economic terms it has a long-term future.
- It is equitable, for instance, it is founded on principles of fairness and justice and does not tolerate discrimination.

As the model in Figure 13.2 outlines, community development workers support individuals to make changes through: developing new skills (*personal empowerment*), working together (*community organisation*) and participating in political structures (*participation and involvement*). Community development has a particular focus on supporting fair and just communities, working in areas of highest deprivation and concentrating on individuals who are traditionally most excluded like those from black and ethnic minorities or people with learning disabilities (*practising positive action*). These working processes make up the four community empowerment dimensions.

The outcomes they seek from their work, and the reason why most community members would get involved, would be to make communities safer,

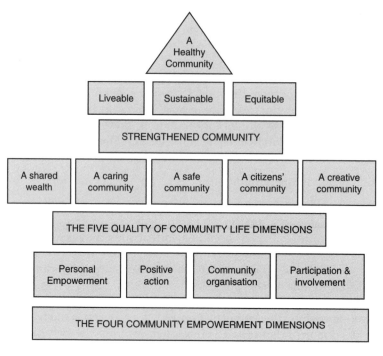

Figure 13.2   Model of community development
Source: Barr and Hashagen (1999) Reprinted with permission from A. Barr and S. Hashagen

more caring, wealthier, more creative and more democratic. These outcomes make up the five quality of community life dimensions (see Figure 13.2).

Accepting this analysis means that community development workers need to become more aware of their responsibilities towards people with learning disabilities in order to support them to overcome the barriers they find within communities. They need to be working with people with learning disabilities, their friends, families and support workers to ensure that they have the opportunity to be included in civic society.

The main drawback of this approach is that it has hardly been tested. For many community development workers, this will be a new and challenging role for which they will need support and training. Training could take place as part of mainstream community development or community education courses, or it could take the form of particular courses around equalities, potentially run by people with learning disabilities themselves. In any case community development workers need to develop a clear picture of how and where people with learning disabilities are living in their localities so that they can enable them to join in particular aspects of that community's life.

Active citizenship

Political interest in participation and citizenship means that there are now workers in the health services, leisure sector, voluntary organisations and Local Strategic Partnerships (Community Planning Partnerships in Scotland), as well as in community education, who are using community development skills and supporting individuals to make a contribution to their communities. In practice, despite their emphasis on the most excluded individuals, most of these workers do not work with people with learning disabilities. They might think that other people like social workers do that. They might think that it takes specially qualified people to work with people with disabilities or they might not understand that people with learning disabilities have gifts to bring to a community.

Promoting inclusive communities and enabling individuals to make an active contribution are supported by government policy:

> *The Government's vision for active communities is of strong, active and empowered communities – increasingly capable of doing things for themselves, defining the problems they face and then tackling them together. It is a vision in which everyone – no matter what their age, race or social background – has a sense of belonging and a stake in society*
> (Home Office, active communities: www.homeoffice.co.uk)

The government Strategy for Neighbourhood Renewal is a scheme for putting more resources into the most deprived communities. Although, again this assesses needs rather than assets, it does mean that there are more resources in these areas, which could be made available to help people with learning disabilities access their community and take up their role as citizens. Some areas employ local people or 'community animateurs' to help promote and organise the participation of community members in activities that help to make positive changes to their community. These people could make very effective 'community guides' in the context of people with learning disabilities. People with learning disabilities need to be encouraged and supported to assert their rights as citizens in localities by using mainstream support and funding to access their community and influence services.

Why should human services professionals adopt a community perspective in their work?

Having considered ways to overcome the barriers faced by people when interacting within their community, it is important to consider why professionals need to consider this as part of their work. Government expectations that people with learning disabilities will participate in community and civic life appear in a number of recent policy documents. For example, the White Paper, *Valuing People* declares: '*Our new agenda needs to be based on social inclusion, civil rights, choice and independence*' (Department of Health 2001: 21). The Green Paper, *Independence, Well-being and Choice*, sets the target that: '*By 2025 disabled people in Britain will be respected as equal members of society*' (Department of Health 2005: 7). These papers acknowledge that, if these expectations are to be met, services must change radically. Many people with learning disabilities are presented with a limited choice of services and these are based on a model that has remained largely unchanged since the 1970s. Figure 13.3 shows a typical Local Authority's expenditure on learning disability services. The vast majority of this authority's spending is committed to group homes, specialist placements (mostly out-of-authority) and day centres. In each of these, disabled people spend their time with groups of other disabled people and staff. Involvement in local communities is often minimal.

This service profile is set to change. Both the White Paper, *Our Health, Our Care, Our Say* (Department of Health 2006) and the Prime Minister's Strategy Unit paper, *Improving the Life Chances of Disabled People* (Cabinet Office 2005) point to the use of individual budgets as the likely cornerstone of social care in the coming years. In 2006/7, the Government tested individual budgets in 13 pilot sites and this work built on the substantial body of knowledge produced through the work of in Control, a partnership which

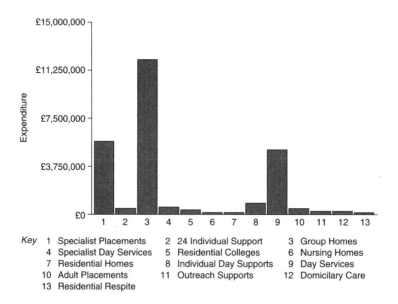

Figure 13.3   One Local Authority's typical expenditure on learning disability services
Source: in Control

continues to develop a new model of social care based on personalised budgets.

The significance of this move, in which disabled people will have control over the planning, arranging and funding of their support, is indicated in the findings of an evaluation of six in Control pilot sites.

In just under a year significant changes were noted in the community participation of 31 people who had taken control of their funding and support.

- All 10 people living in residential care before taking control had moved to their own accommodation within a year.
- Use of day centres dropped an average of one day per person per week.
- Satisfaction with community life overall increased in proportion.
- Eleven people had said that they were unhappy with their social lives at the beginning of the process, just under a year later none of the 31 people said they were unhappy.

(Poll et al. 2006)

These changes were achieved simply because people were able to exercise choice. These outcomes suggest that individuals, once in control of their support, will organise their lives in such ways that they participate more actively in community life.

There is therefore an opportunity for professionals to become more adept at helping people to become involved in communities, to facilitate connections rather than to deliver services that, arguably, are incompatible with community involvement. Judith Snow's assertion that everyone brings a gift to their community leads us to a conclusion that, if this gift is not given, any given community is that much poorer. At a conference in 2002, John McKnight told a story that highlights how professionals can either hold back or facilitate the giving of people's gifts (see Box 13.1).

A switch from a deficit-based model, where people are seen in terms of their needs, to an asset-based approach where people are seen in terms of their gifts and contributions is probably the single greatest change that professionals can make if they are to facilitate rather than block connections to the community, as is demonstrated in the story in Box 13.1.

What professionals can do to enable people to make connections in their communities

If social care professionals are to play a facilitating role in the development of people's community connections, they must examine their own attitude to

---

Box 13.1 The blessing of giving

In Cincinnati a number of churches ran a soup kitchen together. Homeless people came to the basement of a church to eat. As one of the pastors involved was giving a sermon on 'It is more blessed to give than to receive', the thought struck him that he was denying a blessing to the homeless people who came to the soup kitchen – the blessing of giving. The pastors got together and devised a capacity inventory to use with the homeless people. This asked about gifts and skills. One of the questions was: 'If you could start a business, what would you do? What do you like to do that people might pay for?' The answer of the majority was 'I would cook'. (Incidentally, half of the homeless people had had their own business!)

Do you see what the failure to understand the gifts of people is about? Here is a bunch of inept Methodists – two-thirds of them couldn't fry an egg – feeding people whose major talent was cooking.[1]

---

community, as shown in Activity 13.1. Until now most professionals have not needed to consider their own beliefs about community in their working lives. A belief in the hospitality of communities is not part of the person specification in most human service jobs. A job as a support worker helping people with learning disabilities to be 'included' is not necessarily incompatible with a personal view that communities are dead or dangerous.

John McKnight argues that a positive role for paid staff is that of community connector. One of the main attributes of a good community connector is a fundamental belief in community. This belief is based in a positive choice to focus on the good things in the community – an asset-based approach. In practice, this will involve mapping both the gifts of individuals and the assets of the community. Person-centred planning has familiarised many staff with a gifts focus: the identification of the good things about people, their qualities, talents and skills. There are a number of gifts map pro formas. Figure 13.4 is a simple example.

Activity 13.3

Using the gifts map in Figure 13.4, think think about one person you love and care for and write down their list of gifts. Now think about a person you work with who has a learning disability and think about their list of gifts. Was this easy to do? How much were you affected by your professional thinking? How much were you affected by the deficit-based model?

Identity	Gifts
The roles we play in family and the community, for example: husband, father, workmate, member of church.	The unique qualities a person has, for example: makes people laugh, calmness, generosity.
Skills	**Interests**
Specific skills, for example, typing, sewing, cooking, speaking in public.	Hobbies or specific interests: for example: *Star Trek*, gardening, football.

Figure 13.4 Gifts map

For many people, this is difficult to do, though obviously not all of us. If this map is filled out while maintaining a steadfastly positive approach, a refreshing and different view of the person often emerges. This positive approach needs to include a constant questioning of what a deficit is and an attempt to reframe negatives to become positives. In this way 'challenging behaviour' might become 'he really knows how to tell us when things are wrong'. 'Overweight' could become 'food lover'. The cataloguing or collecting interest that some autistic people have might be translated into useful job skills. Success in this area is one of the first steps to understanding the gifts a person can offer their community.

Supporting 'mutual aid'

The importance of knowing what people can contribute is critical if professionals are to help people connect. Young and Lemos (1997) argue that community is a process of exchange, of mutual aid.

> *The first and most humble meaning [of mutual aid] is of more or less simultaneous reciprocity between two people, for example A looks after B when B is ill and B looks after A when A is ill.*
> *The second and less humble meaning is lagged reciprocity . . . Friends and neighbours might help one another . . . with no immediate return, but with strong implicit presumption of help to be returned at an unspecified moment of future need. The third . . . meaning is where mutuality is*

> *multilateral – three ways, or four ways, or multiple ways. A helps B, B helps C, C helps A. This multilateral aid can be stretched to include millions of people who are unknown, but although unknown, contribute to the welfare of each and every one of us.*

The implication here is that, if we are to help people take part in community, it is critical to know what they bring. Our objective in helping people to be part of the community is that they develop relationships. However, if we do not know what they are able to contribute to the community exchange process, there will be an unequal interaction, a one-way process based on charity towards the disabled person.

Mapping communities

Understanding how to map communities is another essential skill for the professional who wants to facilitate community connections. Some mapping techniques are elaborate and painstaking. John McKnight (1997) sets out a series of approaches, for example, in his *Guide to Capacity Inventories*, based on a detailed house-by-house survey.

McKnight shows how the land, the economy, systems (for example, institutions, service organisations and businesses), associations and individuals are the five possible starting points to building a community (see Figure 13.5). He suggests that associations may be the most productive area when thinking of how people with learning disabilities can be involved in communities.

McKnight states that studies carried out by his Institute revealed that, in conscious connection work with excluded groups, 80 per cent of successful community building projects were created through associations. Associations are groups of unpaid people who gather together for a common purpose or interest – perhaps at the karaoke night at the pub, or a group of people concerned about road safety in their street. These may be well organised, such as campaigns, or loose groups such as baby-sitting exchanges or people who gather at a particular pub to go to football matches.

McKnight suggests that associations are important in the context of support work with people with disabilities because it is in associations that people gather for the express purpose of being in a relationship with others. A disabled person who shares the interest of an association has a good chance of being welcomed despite any prejudice on the part of individual association members.

When professionals undertake community mapping, they often begin by locating facilities like the swimming pool or doctor's surgery. While these are important, they are easy to add as the map nears completion. If people are to be supported to find relationships in the community, finding out where

land/resources

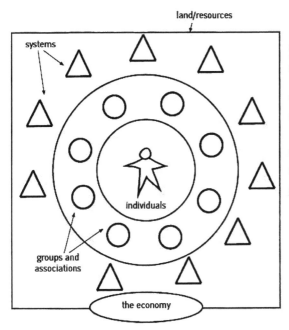

5 building blocks of community

- individuals
- groups and associations
- systems
- land/resources
- the economy

Figure 13.5 The five building blocks of community
Source: As presented by John McKnight in a 2002 Paradigm/KeyRing Conference: From Client To Citizen

associations are should be the starting point. The process of finding out can be a simple one – asking people in the neighbourhood what associations they belong to. In an average metropolitan neighbourhood there will certainly be several hundred and, probably, thousands of associations – potential contact points for people with learning disabilities to make a connection. Having identified the places or associations people can connect with, a structure for supporting this is important. One such structure is a circle of support.

Circles of support

A circle of support is a group of people who gather round an individual to support him or her to make decisions about his or her life and then to help take those decisions forward. Every circle is different, because every individual is different. Some circles start small and grow much larger as new people get invited in. Others start small and stay small. Some circles have long periods of time when they are not used by the focus person but are re-activated at a time of crisis or decision-making, while others meet regularly for years. Most circles are close-knit groups of people, who meet informally with a common purpose around one individual.

Circles sometimes emerge out of the meeting of an existing network, most of the time they are established by one or two people. Commitment is needed to start a circle, initially from one or two people who are standing by the focus person, but soon from everyone involved in the circle. Someone needs to take on the role of facilitator, at least at the first few circle meetings, so that the circle gets off the ground. This may end up being a staff member in the first instance. But it is crucial that the circle is ultimately made of people who voluntarily give their time to support the person. Even if a staff member joins in her own time she might find themselves facing a conflict of interest if the circle needs to take up an issue with the service provider.

Circles can be difficult to get started because they require a high level of commitment and the beginnings of a network to be in place. But when they work well, they can achieve great change and they can provide a fast and safe track to inclusion. Daphne's story illustrates how they can work (see Box 13.2).

Box 13.2 Daphne's circle of support

Daphne is in her early thirties, and very outgoing. She has some support from staff but not all the time. At times when she was not being supported, Daphne would often take herself to the hospital saying she had a broken leg or some other complaint. Liz, an independent facilitator brought in to work with Daphne, thought that she might like a circle of support and asked her about it. Daphne was very keen on the idea but had no one to ask in to her circle. Liz asked one of her support team who invited five of her own relatives and friends. Daphne threw a party for them so that by the time Liz arrived to facilitate the first circle meeting they were all quite merry.

Liz immediately noticed a young woman, Brenda, who was used to chairing meetings and asked her to co-facilitate. The meeting went well because everyone was really enjoying themselves. Daphne talked about wanting to drive a car and get married. Some people present weren't sure what they would have to offer but Liz helped them to see what they could contribute. One woman was a member of a knitting club and she invited Daphne to go along with her. Daphne has met lots of new friends through the knitting club.

After a couple of meetings Liz pulled out, leaving Brenda to facilitate. Since then the circle has doubled in size. It has raised £1000 for a holiday for Daphne, accompanied her to visit her clan in the North of Scotland, gone go-karting with her as a preparation for learning to drive and thrown a 'wedding party' in which everyone dressed up. Daphne is delighted with the effect it has had on her life and is too busy to visit the hospital any more.

The professionals' strategic role in building community

In addition to the very important roles outlined previously, professionals can also have a much more strategic role in building and developing community. In researching this chapter we found some examples of new and exciting initiatives, some led by mainstream services, others by progressive service providers which were overcoming the barriers identified earlier and supporting and enabling people with learning disabilities to be a real part of their communities.

Activity 13.4

Before reading the following exemplars think about any opportunities in your area to connect people with groups who share an interest that enhances the community.

You may have thought about groups that come together to provide an informal support or service to a community, you may have thought of pressure groups or environmental groups. You may have looked at the work of your local People First group and seen them involved in working with organisations such as the criminal justice system. The opportunities are endless, if we choose to let them be. The following exemplars demonstrate how some organisations came together to support the community involvement of some people who have a learning disability.

Sustainable Dialogues

The Sustainable Dialogues initiative in Clackmannanshire is an example of local planning structure where people with learning disabilities have been able to get involved, and a community worker has collaborated with an advocacy worker for people with learning disabilities. The community worker did not deliberately adopt any of the models of practice outlined earlier. However, she did understand that people with learning disabilities were excluded, and that she had a role in supporting them to become more fully involved as citizens in their community. Her awareness might have been enhanced by the happy circumstance of sharing an office with the People First Development Officer, who worked from a social model of disability.

The Voices Group is a branch of People First Scotland, which is based in Clackmannanshire. The community planning officer at the local council for voluntary organisations (CVS) spoke to the group about getting involved in community planning and, as a result of their interest, invited them along to take part. Members of Voices have become involved in Sustainable Dialogues, an environmental forum which feeds directly into the Community Planning process. Other members of Sustainable Dialogues include the local branch of Friends of the Earth, the allotment society, the Credit Union, the police and the local council.

The group meets on a monthly basis to discuss local and national issues of environmental interest and plan what should be done about them in Clackmannanshire. Their views are passed on to the environmental subgroup of the Community Planning Partnership. The members of the Voices group were made welcome from the start. The atmosphere is friendly and relaxed and everyone's contribution is respected. Sustainable Dialogues have now adopted a system of meetings management, which was originally developed by People First and is now used in many different forums. An individual who does not understand the jargon or who has missed the point of what is being said holds up a red card. An individual who wants to speak holds up a green card. In this way the chair of the meeting can ensure that everyone is following what is happening and that everyone gets a chance to make a contribution. The community planning officer thinks it is a 'fantastic tool which promotes inclusion'. The cards enable everyone to feel more comfortable and speak up when they do not understand what is going on.

As a result of her participation in Sustainable Dialogues, Mary from the Voices group was invited to the housing forum. Her contribution was much appreciated and that forum has also adopted the red and green card system. This initiative was based on collaboration between a community development worker and a support worker for people with learning disabilities. The support worker was willing to enable those she supports to take some risks by getting involved, while the community development worker did not see people with learning disabilities as 'someone else's problem'. The presence of the people with learning disabilities themselves within the Sustainable Dialogues group, overcame any fear, hostility or prejudice which might have existed.

Quality Action Group

The Quality Action Group in Stirling is another example of how an effective partnership between voluntary sector providers and mainstream services can support people with learning disabilities to have a real voice in their locality. It started in 1993 as an initiative run by the then Scottish Office and two voluntary sector providers aimed at promoting the inclusion of people with learning disabilities in Stirling: '*Many of us found that being in a community is not the same as being part of it. We needed to find ways that we could be included.*'[2]

One member of staff was seconded to the project to meet with the managers of mainstream leisure facilities to discuss how people with learning disabilities could be included more effectively. It soon became clear that people with learning disabilities themselves needed to meet the service managers. A group was formed and one of their first activities was a tour of local community centres.

The group aimed to make changes in the way that they were treated, both by services and by the community at large. It attracted funding from a range of sources and is now managed by a committee of 23 adults with learning disabilities, supported by Key Housing and Stirling Council Community Services. The group employs its own staff and combines providing services, with lobbying on behalf of people with learning disabilities at a local and national level.

Members of the group have taken part in a variety of local initiatives including environmental campaigns. They provide awareness raising and training sessions for youth groups, local schools, the police and local council employees as part of their drive to change attitudes.

They also maintain close links with community learning and development staff. They are directly involved in a local Community Learning Plan for People with Learning Disabilities and are frequently asked to comment on council plans and strategies.

The group has provided an opportunity for personal growth. Individuals who started out scared to voice an opinion and struggling to manage their money have learnt to chair meetings and to manage large budgets. It has also enabled people with learning disabilities to contribute to their community both through getting involved in local campaigns and through actively contributing to local service plans.

As in the Sustainable Dialogues initiative, those who started the project did not consciously adopt a particular model of practice. Instead they responded directly to the expressed needs of people with learning disabilities. However, the community development workers involved understood their role in supporting people with learning disabilities as excluded members of their communities. The support workers and the people with learning disabilities themselves were willing to take the risks of getting to know their community, in the way described by John McKnight, and getting involved in local community life. In this way, they too overcame the barriers of fear, hostility and prejudice.

Grapevine

Grapevine is an organisation based in Coventry, which seeks to empower people with learning disabilities and support them to be full members of their communities. It bases much of its practice on the models developed by Judith Snow and John McKnight. Particular efforts have been made to overcome barriers such as staff ignorance of the local community by employing local staff or supporting them to get to know the community. Both staff and people who use the service, are willing to take the risk of getting involved and combating prejudice.

As an organisation, Grapevine has tried hard to get involved in local planning structures to enable the people it supports to have a voice. One person with learning disabilities is supported to be the 'equalities champion' for the equalities theme group of the Local Strategic Partnership. Grapevine also has a representative on the steering group of the local Community Empowerment Network. The Network holds quarterly events for up to 350 local organisations and individuals and, while a staff member represents Grapevine, an individual with learning disabilities goes along as a community member in his own right. The Network also has a 'marketplace' on its website which Grapevine uses to post up opportunities for connection.

Grapevine was awarded a grant by the Local Strategic Partnership for its campaign against hate crime targeted at people with learning disabilities. People with learning disabilities involved in that campaign have now joined the steering group of the city-wide Hate Crime Reduction Partnership, which works with all 'at risk' groups. Grapevine is currently working with the Regional Assembly to try to ensure that what it has learnt about hate crime is built into future reduction strategies.

Grapevine also supports people to become part of their communities in more informal ways. It organises and hosts a local community festival and gives grants to people with learning disabilities to develop their own ideas. Some young people have been running regular club nights at a local pub, which are open to anyone who wants to come along.

Although Grapevine is now well known in the local community and the people it supports are beginning to have their voice heard and build new connections, the organisation feels that there is a long way to go. Mainstream agencies are not knocking at the door asking to include people with learning disabilities and Grapevine is continuing to work hard to have their voices heard. Currently the organisation is working to develop city-wide standards for involving people with learning disabilities which, it hopes, will go further towards protecting their rights as citizens.

Small Sparks

Small Sparks is a small grants programme tested by in Control as a practical, inexpensive means of helping people to get involved. The name and idea of Small Sparks are borrowed from the successful community development project run by the City of Seattle Department of Neighbourhoods, 'Involve all Neighbours Project'.[3]

Four local authorities received £2,500 from in Control to distribute as grants of up to £250 on a match-funding basis. Small Sparkers could provide their contribution in funding (perhaps got as a donation from a local business), in materials or volunteer labour.

There were simple criteria for the projects:

- they must involve new people in the neighbourhood;
- they must be completed within eight weeks;
- a record must be made (probably in photos);
- Small Sparkers must come and tell their story at a celebration.

The local authorities had to ensure that the programme remained low tech, low administration and low scrutiny – trusting people to use the £250 sensibly. In practice, this meant that local authorities handed over the funds in cash and then waited to see what happened. There was minimal worker involvement.

Any fears that funds might be misused or wasted proved to be unfounded. People, without exception, used their Small Sparks grants responsibly.

For this very small investment (both in funds and in the minimal worker input required) 40 diverse and imaginative projects were produced. They included celebrating the 30th anniversary of a local toy library, under-5's sports day, Easy Steps to Banking (in which disabled people explained the right to hold a bank account in a local bank), a barbecue to bring local allotment holders together (so that the people with a learning disablity could meet their fellow gardeners). In each of these cases, the disabled people were seen not as people getting a service, but leaders of a community project which was useful for other local people.

Each at least doubled the £250 investment with the matching of resources from the Small Sparker. One project, a sponsored cycle ride, produced a £7,000 return for a local charity.

The modest amount of funding involved in Small Sparks might suggest that this approach is peripheral to any strategic approach to community involvement. This is, though, a practical tool which could be at the centre of a strategy for inclusion and, particularly, prevention.

The grants can be offered to anyone – including those people with high support needs. But they are of particular interest for those people who are on the edge of eligibility for a social service. Currently, some people who are not eligible for services may fare badly when isolated and left to their own resources. For want of a little support these people can find themselves on a downward spiral of problems – possibly leading towards crisis and, ironically, eligibility for services. This is a scenario well known to many social services staff. *Independence, Well-being and Choice* supports the approach exemplified by Small Sparks: '*There is a small but growing evidence base indicating significant potential benefits in low-level prevention aiming at improving well-being*' (Department of Health 2005: 3).

Small Sparks projects work best when not launched from within care group silos. Those projects which reach out to find allies within the community produce perhaps the most enduring results – relationships which extend beyond the life of the project. Finding local people who share an interest and want to jointly organise the project seems key to an integrated community development approach.

Conclusion

In this chapter we have explored a wide range of contributions that professionals can make to support people who have a learning disability to become valued members of their community. This has included an exposition of the approaches that are useful when considering ways to build community and their helpfulness in overcoming some of the barriers we are very familiar with. We have also discussed the ways in which you as professionals can work with individuals to help them make connections within their community and strategic challenges that we can contribute to in order to make the sea change from communities that do not include people who have a learning disability to one that does so and does so willingly and on an equal basis. In achieving this a switch from a deficit-based, where people are seen in terms of their needs, to an asset-based approach where people are seen in terms of their gifts and contributions is probably the single greatest change that professionals can make if they are to facilitate rather than block connections to community. In a nutshell, this involves:

- using person centred practice to really get to know the person and appreciate their gifts;
- working out what the person might want from a connection;
- mapping the community, and the person's networks to begin to see where the opportunities might lie;
- introducing the person to other people, really focusing on their gifts and what she or he has to offer;
- supporting the person to maintain his or her friendships through keeping in touch and reciprocating whenever possible;
- supporting the person with any new emotions which develop through the friendship.

Notes

1   John McKnight, speech at Making the Community Connection, Paradigm/ KeyRing, 2000.
2   A Quality Action Group member quoted in *The Chance for Us to Change Things*, an information booklet by Stirling Quality Action Group.
3   www.ci.seattle.wa.us/neighborhoods/involve/

Annotated bibliography

Kennedy, J., Sanderson, H. and Wilson, H. (2002) *Friendship and Community: Practical Strategies for Making Connections in Communities*. Manchester: North West Training and Development Team.
A book aimed at those who support people with learning disabilities and their families to help them work towards inclusion. There are chapters covering person centred planning, developing networks, mapping your community and making a contribution. Many of the strategies in the book are equally applicable to anyone excluded from community life.

ARK Community Networks (2006) *Community Matters: Taking Action and Making a Difference in your Local Community. A Training Pack for Promoting Active Citizenship*.
The training course is aimed at people with learning disabilities. It is designed to enhance understanding and facilitate learning about Citizenship, Democracy, the structures and opportunities within Community Planning (Local Strategic Partnerships) and how people can be more active in their communities about issues that concern them. It suggests activities, session plans and handouts which might be useful in addressing these issues. (ARK Community Networks, The Priory, Canaan Lane, Edinburgh EH10 4SG).

Schwartz, D. (1992) *Who Cares? Rediscovering Community*. New Haven, CT: Westview Press. (UK distributor: Values Incorporated).
This book contains an analysis of why people with learning disabilities are excluded from community and stories of inclusion.

References

Barr, A. and Hashagen, S. (1999) *Achieving Better Community Development*. Manchester: CDF.
Cabinet Office (2005) *Improving the Life Chances of Disabled People*. London: Stationery Office.
Department of Health (2001) *Valuing People: A New Strategy for Learning Disability for the 21st Century*. London: Department of Health.
Department of Health (2005) *Independence Well-being and Choice: Our Vision for the Future of Social Care for Adults in England*. London: Stationery Office.
Department of Health (2006) *Our Health, Our Care, Our Say*. London: Stationery Office.
Jones, C. (1998) The meaning of community care for people with learning difficulties and paid support staff, unpublished MSc thesis.

Kennedy, J., Sanderson, H. and Wilson, H. (2002) *Friendship and Community: Practical Strategies for Making Connections in Communities*. Manchester: North West Training and Development Team.

Lee, D. and Newby, H. (1983) *The Problem of Sociology: An Introduction to the Discipline*. London: Unwin Hyman.

McKnight, J. (1996) *The Careless Society*. New York, Basic Books.

McKnight, J. (1997) A Guide to Capacity Inventories: Mobilising the Community Skills of Local Residents. Chicago.

Oliver, M. (1990) *The Politics of Disablement*. London: Macmillan Press.

Poll, C., Duffy, S., Hatton, C., Sanderson, H. and Routledge, M. (2006) *A Report on in Control's First Phase 2003–2005*. London: in Control Publications.

Putnam, R.D. (2001) *Bowling Alone: The Collapse and Revival of the American Community*. New York: Simon & Schuster.

Scottish Executive (2000) *Same as You: A Review of the Services for People with a Learning Disability*. Edinburgh: Scottish Executive.

Snow, J. (1994) *What's Really Worth Doing and How to Do it*. Toronto: Inclusion Press.

The Stationery Office (2004) *The Disability Discrimination Act*. London.

Young, M. and Lemos, G. (1997) *The Communities We Have Lost and Can Regain*. London: Environment and Planning.

Useful resources

City of Seattle website
www.ci.seattle.wa.us

For information about the Disability Discrimination Act
www.direct.gov.uk

For more information about asset-based community development
www.northwestern.edu/ipr/abcd

For further information of the Doncaster Health Action Zone community animateurs
www.sccd.org.uk/reports/hazg.doc

Index

Related books from Open University Press
Purchase from www.openup.co.uk or order through your local bookseller

---

INTELLECTUAL DISABILITY
SOCIAL APPROACHES
David Race

This could have been a triumphant book; instead it is a sober one, and far more useful for it . . . Based on an around-the-world tour of countries where the concepts of normalization and Social Role Valorization have been influential, the book offers a comparative account of the ways these ideas have worked out in seven different national contexts more than thirty years after their introduction.

From the Foreword by John O'Brien,
The Centre on Human Policy, Syracuse University, USA

- How do services in different countries vary across the lifespan?
- What lessons can the different countries learn from one another?

Based on the author's own experience from over thirty years in the field, this thought-provoking book offers a comparative study of services for people with intellectual disabilities in seven countries: England, Australia, Canada, New Zealand, Norway, Sweden and the USA. Through the author's discussions with people with intellectual disabilities, parents and families, and those involved with services at a professional and academic level, the book provides a critical reflection on intellectual disability services across the lifespan.

Each chapter contains the following key features:

- A brief 'Instant Impacts' reflection of an incident or a person encountered in the country concerned
- A short history of services in the country and a summary of the current service system
- A detailed look at services through the age range, including issues around screening and pre-birth
- Drawing on the author's own experience of being a parent of a child with intellectual disabilities, 'Adam's World Tour' boxes include a summary of the author's views on the likely services Adam might receive in the country concerned

Intellectual Disability is key reading for students of social work, learning disability nursing, social policy and community work, as well as those training to work with people with intellectual disabilities in health and social care services. Because of its unique approach, however, it is as relevant to families of people with intellectual disabilities as it is to professionally qualified practitioners and policy makers.

Contents
Foreword – Acknowledgements – Dedication – Introduction: A personal approach – Demographic Overview – Sweden: Rational, orderly, enjoyable and healthy lives? – Norway: Big brother's shadow or going the extra mile? – New Zealand: A values led market? – Australia: Who pays; who cares? – Canada: Values still to the fore? – The United States of America: Freedom to roam the jungle? – England: Home and beauty? – Last thoughts, hopes and fears – References

2007   288pp

ISBN: 978 0 335 22136 3 (Paperback)
ISBN: 978 0 335 22137 0 (Hardback)

LEARNING DISABILITY
A LIFE CYCLE APPROACH TO VALUING PEOPLE

Gordon Grant, Peter Goward, Malcolm Richardson and Paul Ramcharan

This practical and accessible key text examines the nature and impact of collaboration between different professional and voluntary groups working together to deliver services. The first section explores partnership in terms of language, politics, diversity, user perspectives, rurality and ethics. In section two, carefully selected authors draw upon their expertise to raise key questions, and use case studies to demonstrate the challenges of working in partnership in areas where collaboration is a crucial to effective practice, this includes: child protection; drug using parents; dementia; travelling families; domestic violence; learning difficulties; homelessness; mentally disordered offenders; HIV and AIDS; disaffected youth and older people.

This book is recommended reading for managers, practitioners and students from a variety of human service agencies – it will provide good understanding into issues, pitfalls and best practice to work effectively in partnership with other agencies. A must read for anyone about to develop or join a multi-agency partnership.

Contributors
Althea Allison; John Bates; Liz Blyth; Julian Buchanan; Ros Carnwell; Alex Carson; Pat Chambers; Michael Clark; Brian Corby; Jacquie Evans; Ian Iles; David Jolley; Thoby Miller; Amir Minhas; Virginia Minogue; Neil Moreland; Lester Parrott; Judith Phillips; Richard Pugh; Kate Read; Angela Roberts; Debbie Williams; Ruth Wilson; Ruth Wyner

Contents
Acknowledgements – About the Editors – List of Contributors – Preface – Part One: The Construction of Learning Disability – Part Two: Childhood: Rights, Risks and Responsibilities – Part Three: Independence: Adolescents and the Younger Adult – Part Four: Social Inclusion and Adulthood – Part Five: Citizenship and the Older Adult – Index

2005   784pp
ISBN-13: 978 0 335 21439 6 (ISBN-10: 0 335 21439 8) Paperback
ISBN-13: 978 0 335 21864 4 (ISBN-10: 0 335 21826 1) Hardback